Protecting Children from Domestic Violence

Protecting Children from Domestic Violence

Strategies for Community Intervention

Edited by
PETER G. JAFFE
LINDA L. BAKER
ALISON J. CUNNINGHAM

THE GUILFORD PRESS
New York   London

© 2004 The Guilford Press
A Division of Guilford Publications, Inc.
72 Spring Street, New York, NY 10012
www.guilford.com

Printed in the United States of America

This book is printed on acid-free paper.

Last digit is print number: 9 8 7 6 5 4 3 2 1

Library of Congress Cataloging-in-Publication Data

Protecting children from domestic violence : strategies for community
intervention / [edited by] Peter G. Jaffe, Linda L. Baker, Alison J.
Cunningham.
     p. cm.
Includes bibliographical references and index.
   ISBN 1-57230-992-X (cloth : alk. paper)
  1. Family violence—United States. 2. Family violence—Canada. 3. Child
abuse—United States—Prevention. 4. Child abuse—Canada—Prevention.
5. Family services—United States. 6. Family services—Canada. I. Jaffe,
Peter G. II. Baker, Linda L. III. Cunningham, Alison J.
   HV6626.2.P76 2004
   362.82′9256—dc22

                                                       2003025661

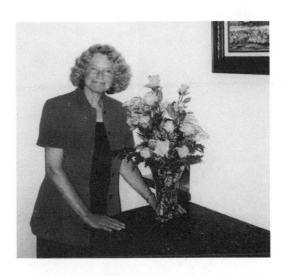

This book is dedicated to our friend and colleague Robbie Rossman, whom we lost tragically in May 2002. She was an inspiration to all of us for her energy, intellect, and insights as a researcher, mentor, and clinician. We miss her warm smile, her encouragement and support, and her joy for living. She leaves a legacy of understanding and community action on behalf of children and families in crisis.

About the Editors

Peter G. Jaffe, PhD, is Special Advisor on Violence Prevention and was the Founding Director of the Centre for Children and Families in the Justice System of the London Family Court Clinic, a children's mental health center specializing in issues that bring children and families into the justice system. Dr. Jaffe is a clinical adjunct professor in the Department of Psychology and Psychiatry at the University of Western Ontario, and is on the faculty of the National Council of Juvenile and Family Court Judges Family Violence Department's "Enhancing Judicial Skills in Domestic Violence Cases" workshops. In 1980, he was the founding Chairperson of the London Coordinating Committee to End Woman Abuse and has been actively involved in research on the impact of domestic violence on children. He has also been involved in provincial and national panels examining the issue of domestic violence and currently is a member of the Domestic Violence Death Review Committee, established by Ontario's Chief Coroner. Dr. Jaffe has coauthored several books on domestic violence, including *Children of Battered Women, Working Together to End Domestic Violence,* and *Child Custody and Domestic Violence: A Call for Safety and Accountability,* and has been instrumental in promoting and developing violence prevention programs in his school district as a trustee for the past 23 years.

Linda L. Baker, PhD, is Executive Director of the Centre for Children and Families in the Justice System of the London Family Court Clinic, and is an adjunct professor in both the Department of Psychology and the Faculty of Education at the University of Western Ontario. Dr. Baker coauthored *Seeking Best Evidence,* a comprehensive review of literature on children who live in homes in which their mothers are abused, for the National Crime Prevention Centre in Canada. Since 1997, she has coauthored over 18 resources to enhance understanding and intervention with children and adolescents, including *Children Exposed to Violence: A Handbook for Police Trainers to Increase Understanding and Improve Community Responses* and *Understanding the Effects of Domestic Violence: A Handbook and Training Manual for Early Childhood Educators.* Dr. Baker has been invited to speak and facilitate workshops in her areas of expertise throughout Canada and the United States.

Alison J. Cunningham, MA, is Director of Research and Planning at the Centre for Children and Families in the Justice System of the London Family Court Clinic. She recently served as Acting Director of the Centre for Research on Violence Against Women and Children, a cooperative venture of the London Coordinating Committee to End Woman Abuse, Fanshawe College, and the University of Western Ontario. She ran a multisite randomized trial of multisystemic therapy for high-risk young offenders, with Dr. Alan Leschied, and is the coauthor, with Curt Griffiths, of two textbooks, *Canadian Criminal Justice: A Primer* and *Canadian Corrections,* as well as author of a number of articles on a wide range of criminal justice topics. She is a member of the London Coordinating Committee to End Woman Abuse and serves on the High-Risk Offender Advisory Board of the London Police and the Advisory Board of the London Community Parole Project, Correctional Service of Canada. She is also President of the Ontario Council of Elizabeth Fry Societies, and in 2001 was invited to be an advisor to the World Health Organization about standards of health services for child and adult victims of sexual violence.

Contributors

Linda L. Baker, PhD, Centre for Children and Families in the Justice System, London Family Court Clinic, London, Ontario, Canada

Nicholas Bala, LLM, Faculty of Law, Queen's University, Kingston, Ontario, Canada

Lundy Bancroft, BA, private practice, Northampton, Massachusetts

Miriam Berkman, JD, MSW, Child Study Center, Yale University, New Haven, Connecticut

Steven J. Berkowitz, MD, Child Study Center, Yale University, New Haven, Connecticut

Jacquelyn Boggess, JD, The Center for Fathers, Families, and Public Policy, Madison, Wisconsin

Perry M. Butterfield, MA, University of Colorado Health Sciences Center, University of Colorado Hospital, Denver, Colorado

Jacquelyn C. Campbell, PhD, School of Nursing, Johns Hopkins University, Baltimore, Maryland

Janet Carter, MA, Family Violence Prevention Fund, San Francisco, California

Robert L. Casey, PhD, Child Study Center, Yale University, New Haven, Connecticut

Claire Crooks, PhD, Department of Psychology, University of Western Ontario, London, Ontario, Canada

Alison J. Cunningham, MA, Centre for Children and Families in the Justice System, London Family Court Clinic, London, Ontario, Canada

Diane L. Davis, MA, LP, Domestic Abuse Project, Minneapolis, Minnesota

Billie Lee Dunford-Jackson, JD, Family Violence Department, National Council of Juvenile and Family Court Judges, Reno, Nevada

Jeffrey L. Edleson, PhD, Minnesota Center Against Violence and Abuse, School of Social Work, University of Minnesota, St. Paul, Minnesota

Sandra A. Graham-Bermann, PhD, Department of Psychology, and Women's Studies Program, University of Michigan, Ann Arbor, Michigan

Hilda M. Halabu, MA, Department of Psychology, University of Michigan, Ann Arbor, Michigan

Jennifer L. Hardesty, PhD, Department of Human and Community Development, University of Illinois at Urbana–Champaign, Champaign, Illinois

Ray Hughes, MEd, Thames Valley District School Board, London, Ontario, Canada

Peter G. Jaffe, PhD, Centre for Children and Families in the Justice System, London Family Court Clinic, London, Ontario, Canada

Melpa Kamateros, MS, The Shield of Athena Family Services, Montreal, Quebec, Canada

Steven Marans, PhD, Child Study Center, Yale University, New Haven, Connecticut

Jacqueline G. Rea, MA, Department of Psychology, University of Denver, Denver, Colorado

B. B. Robbie Rossman, PhD (deceased), formerly at Department of Psychology, University of Denver, Denver, Colorado

Martha Shaffer, LLM, Faculty of Law, University of Toronto, Toronto, Ontario, Canada

Jay G. Silverman, PhD, Harvard School of Public Health, Harvard University, Boston, Massachusetts

Oliver J. Williams, PhD, School of Social Work, University of Minnesota, St. Paul, Minnesota

David Wolfe, PhD, Department of Psychology, University of Western Ontario, London, Ontario, Canada

Acknowledgments

This volume would not have been possible without the support and encouragement of our Centre's dedicated staff and board members. The Centre for Children and Families in the Justice System of the London Family Court Clinic promotes safer communities by integrating research and practice. This lofty vision guides our work and our commitment to children exposed to domestic violence. We benefit from a dynamic work environment where people are not afraid to ask difficult questions and look for a better way to serve the families who come through our doors seeking solutions to complex challenges with which they struggle.

Although our names appear on the cover of this book, this work reflects a great deal of collaboration within our organization and among the contributors and their host agencies and universities. We must single out Karen Rhiger, the Centre's Director of Corporate Services, for her tireless work and organizational skills. She is an incredible resource for fundraising and conference planning who allows us to network across the world. This volume is a reflection of that work.

The Centre gratefully acknowledges the financial support of the Ontario Trillium Foundation, an agency of the Ministry of Tourism, Culture and Recreation. With $100 million in annual funding from the province's charitable gaming initiative, the Foundation provides grants to eligible charitable and not-for-profit organizations in the arts, culture, sports, recreation, environment, and social service sectors. Their grant ensures that libraries across Ontario will have this publication available.

Much of the inspiration for this volume came from the 2001 International Conference on Children Exposed to Domestic Violence held in

London, Ontario, Canada. Almost 1,000 people came together from most Canadian provinces and U.S. states as well as 14 other countries to focus on the plight of abused women and children. That conference would not have been possible without funding from the Packard Foundation, the National Crime Prevention Centre (Department of Justice), and the Ontario Ministry of Community, Family and Children's Services. Lucy Carter of Packard and Patricia Begin of the NCPC were especially helpful in bringing together the diverse groups of people from many parts of the world that made the conference an inspiration.

The three of us, as always, have toiled long hours into the evening and weekend where there were no clocks to punch other than borrowing time from our families. We thank for their forbearance, yet again, and respectfully ask the following people for their forgiveness: Deb, Adam, Aaron, Daniel, Michael, Ed, James, and Hilary.

PETER G. JAFFE
LINDA L. BAKER
ALISON J. CUNNINGHAM

Contents

Protecting Children from Domestic Violence

Part I

INTRODUCTION TO THE PROBLEM

1

Purpose and Overview

PETER G. JAFFE, LINDA L. BAKER, and ALISON J. CUNNINGHAM

From a historical perspective, domestic violence services and innovative practices have developed dramatically. The first North American shelters for abused women opened their doors less than 30 years ago. It was only 20 years ago that the issue was raised in the Canadian parliament by MP Margaret Mitchell, to a chorus of inappropriate comments ("Do you beat your wife, Charlie?") and laughter. The laughter has stopped and been replaced by a clear commitment by all levels of government as well as the general public that domestic violence is a serious criminal and social problem.

The initial progress in the field of domestic violence was in public awareness, police and court responses, and services for victims and perpetrators. More recently, there is an increasing focus on the plight of children exposed to domestic violence. Major conferences and publications in the past decade document the impact of domestic violence on some children's emotional, cognitive, and behavioral adjustment at different stages of development (e.g., Jaffe, Wolfe, & Wilson, 1990; Geffner, Jaffe, & Sudermann, 2000; Graham-Bermann & Edleson, 2001; Groves, 2002). Awareness about the special needs of abused women and their children sparked a tremendous level of research, intervention, prevention, policy, and legislative advances. The fact that children's issues reached unparalleled heights in public consciousness was reflected by the Ontario government's May 9, 2002, speech from the throne, which included the following words:

> Every year, thousands of children see violence in their houses. These children are at risk and often continue a legacy of family violence themselves. Your government will continue to help children who are trapped in violent family situations.

The idea for this book evolved from the 2001 International Conference on Children Exposed to Domestic Violence held in London, Ontario, Canada. Almost 1,000 people from Canada, the United States, as well as 14 other countries, gathered to focus on the plight of abused women and children. The volume is dedicated to expanding our understanding and community collaboration in responding to children and their parents in homes where domestic violence takes place, and it addresses the following three themes: First and foremost, we must find effective ways to end domestic violence to eliminate the tragic toll of lives and human suffering associated with it. Second, successful interventions must address not only the needs of children but also their parents, who are the adult victims and perpetrators. Strategies that see children as independent from their parents will fail to offer meaningful safety and healing interventions. As a third theme, we searched for "promising practices" to recognize the reality that there is insufficient research and evaluation to definitively conclude what is "best." We acknowledge our progress with an optimistic caution that we have many gaps in knowing which community responses are most effective in helping children and their parents end the violence in their lives.

This volume is divided into three parts. The first part focuses on critical issues in successful interventions with children. The second part examines current thinking on interventions with adult victims and perpetrators. Examining the responses of the justice system and human services to children exposed to violence is the theme of the third part. Finally, we offer a concluding chapter to share our ideas about future directions in this field.

OVERVIEW OF THE CHAPTERS

In Chapter 2, Jeffrey L. Edleson addresses the important question of whether children exposed to domestic violence should be deemed to be in need of protection by the state. He argues that, based on the literature and the dreadful experiences of his home state, Minnesota, there can be more harm than good done by this legislative and policy change. He outlines a cautious and reasoned approach that demands a broad array of voluntary services for both children and their mothers and that recognizes the differential impact of domestic violence and the diverse range of circumstances in these families.

In Chapter 3, the late B. B. Robbie Rossman (to whom this book is dedicated) and her colleagues outline their thoughts on the best assessment approaches for young children exposed to domestic violence. This chapter highlights an overlooked population, since many agencies counsel older children and adolescents who have the language to describe the impact of domestic violence. Younger children may exhibit the trauma in ways that require differential assessment and intervention strategies.

In Chapter 4, Diane L. Davis describes her pioneering work in developing group intervention programs for adolescents. As police, communities, and the courts recognize that domestic violence is often exhibited in adolescent relationships as "dating violence," there is a need to have programs like the one Diane Davis outlines for this population. The model as well as some of the critical issues in the intake and assessment process is described.

In Chapter 5, Sandra A. Graham-Bermann and Hilda M. Halabu from the University of Michigan discuss an often ignored topic: making our interventions culturally relevant. Based on their model program for children exposed to domestic violence, the authors illustrate how practitioners may have to rethink the "one-size-fits-all" approach for children. In giving examples of their clinical challenges, the authors raise issues for all of us to consider when intervening with children from diverse cultural backgrounds.

Chapters 6 and 7 address the critical issues of safety planning and risk assessment in domestic violence cases. In Chapter 6, Jennifer L. Hardesty at the University of Illinois at Urbana–Champaign and Jacquelyn C. Campbell of Johns Hopkins University review the importance of safety planning for abused women and their children. Building on the development of the "Danger Assessment Scale," the authors delineate the role that children can play in their own safety planning. Chapter 7 expands this theme by exploring the risks that batterers may pose for their partners and children. Lundy Bancroft and Jay G. Silverman, from Boston, summarize key elements from their recent book entitled *The Batterer as Parent* (Bancroft & Silverman, 2002). The authors point out that in our focus on perpetrators of domestic violence as spouses, we ignore, at the children's peril, the harm engendered by them as parents in both subtle and direct ways.

Chapter 8 offers a positive view of the need to offer rehabilitation to abusers, not only as spouses but also as parents. Oliver J. Williams from the University of Minnesota and his colleagues Jacquelyn Boggess (The Center for Fathers, Families, and Public Policy, Madison, Wisconsin), and Janet Carter (Family Violence Prevention Fund, San Francisco, California) build on the existing fathering movement to encourage men to play an active and nurturing role in their children's lives. The authors argue that all too often fathers' roles are ignored or dismissed in the face of the reality that many men want to change their traditional roles. Some abusers can be engaged in interventions that link their childhood to the childhood they are creating for their children.

In Chapter 9, Melpa Kamateros continues this theme by profiling her innovative programs in Montreal that provide outreach services to various ethnic communities. She and her colleagues at The Shield of Athena Family Services developed creative strategies to ensure that new Canadians recognize the harm inherent in domestic violence and the importance of reaching out to appropriate community services.

In Chapter 10, Miriam Berkman, Robert L. Casey, Steven J. Berkowitz, and Steven Marans profile their innovative program bridging Yale's Child Study Center and the New Haven, Connecticut, police. The authors remind us that the police play an essential role in responding to children traumatized by domestic violence. Through case illustrations and a literature review, they delineate the unique opportunity for partnerships between police and mental health professionals in helping these children and families in crisis.

Chapter 11 examines the family court response to domestic violence in the context of child custody disputes. Martha Shaffer from the University of Toronto and Nicholas Bala from Queen's University provide a Canadian legal perspective on how the courts are beginning to recognize that perpetrators of domestic violence may not be appropriate custodial parents and may require supervised visitation. Based on a review of recently reported cases, the authors conclude that the Canadian family courts are making slow progress in recognizing the plight of children exposed to domestic violence, similar to advances in the United States, Australia, and New Zealand.

Similarly, in Chapter 12, Billie Lee Dunford-Jackson examines the family court system from an American perspective. Specifically, she reviews the varied legislative approaches undertaken by numerous states to address the issue of children exposed to domestic violence, with the goal of protecting children from harm. Billie Lee emphasizes that many of the proposed legislative changes are ineffective because the various levels of government fail to communicate with one another and coordinate services. She concludes that formulating beneficial interventions requires avoiding the "one-size-fits-all" approach and instead acknowledging that every family, situation, and set of needs is different.

Chapter 13 summarizes the potential role of the school system in preventing domestic violence. The five authors represent a collaboration of the Centre for Children and Families in the Justice System, the University of Western Ontario, and the Thames Valley District School Board. The authors offer a blueprint for schools to be more proactive in addressing violence prevention efforts and recommend that healthy relationships become the fourth "R" for the education system. The authors challenge schools to be active partners in ending domestic violence by effective early intervention, innovative curriculum, and community collaboration in prevention.

Chapter 14 affords the editors an opportunity to outline our conclusions from the diverse chapters in this volume. We formulate our ideas in a synopsis of future directions in this rapidly developing field.

We trust this book will have a special place in the library of practitioners and policymakers, helping them to consider some of the far-reaching implications of children's exposure to domestic violence. We feel assured that readers will be challenged and stimulated to build on the existing knowledge base to develop better community responses for these children. We believe that we are at a critical juncture, when tremendous change is possible in how we consider domestic violence and its inevitable harm on children and the ripple effects it has on our communities.

REFERENCES

Bancroft, L., & Silverman, J. (2002). *The batterer as parent: Addressing the impact of domestic violence on family dynamics.* Thousand Oaks, CA: Sage.

Geffner, R. A., Jaffe, P. G., & Sudermann, M. (2000). *Children exposed to domestic violence.* New York: Haworth Press.

Graham-Bermann, S. A., & Edleson, J. L. (2001). *Domestic violence in the lives of children.* Washington, DC: American Psychological Association.

Groves, B. (2002). *Children who see too much.* Boston: Beacon Press.

Jaffe, P. G., Wolfe, D. A., & Wilson, S. (1990). *Children of battered women.* Newbury Park, CA: Sage.

2

Should Childhood Exposure to Adult Domestic Violence Be Defined as Child Maltreatment under the Law?

JEFFREY L. EDLESON

The issues of child maltreatment and adult domestic violence have separately received extensive public attention over the past three decades. Yet it is only in the past 10 years that children who are exposed to domestic violence but not themselves victims of abuse have been identified and extensively studied. Several recent research reviews reveal that many children exposed to adult domestic violence may experience a variety of negative developmental outcomes, and may also be at risk for direct physical abuse (Appel & Holden, 1998; Edleson, 1999a, 1999b; Fantuzzo & Mohr, 1999; Margolin, 1998; O'Leary, Slep, & O'Leary, 2000; Rossman, 2001).

A heated national debate is emerging around the question of whether children exposed to adult domestic violence should be defined as maltreated. Some of these emerging efforts are creating unintended negative consequences for families and the systems serving them. This chapter first reviews the research on childhood exposure to adult domestic violence, the variability of children's experiences, and emerging laws aimed at protecting these children. The chapter then makes an argument against assuming that childhood exposure to violence is automatically a form of child maltreatment, and suggests the need for redesigning child protection services and expanding unique, community-based voluntary responses to these children and their families.

ESTIMATES OF CHILDREN'S EXPOSURE

Estimates of the number of children in the United States who are exposed to adult domestic violence each year vary greatly and are based mostly on extrapolating figures from national surveys. It is estimated that many millions of American children are exposed to domestic violence each year. These estimates may be even higher, depending on the samples studied (see Edleson, 1999b; Fantuzzo & Mohr, 1999; Jouriles, McDonald, Norwood, & Ezell, 2001). The incidence of exposure will be discussed in more detail in Chapter 3. What is less clear is what impact such exposure has on individual children.

IMPACT OF VIOLENCE EXPOSURE ON CHILDREN

Almost a hundred published studies report associations between exposure to domestic violence and current child problems or later adult problems. Only about one-third of these studies separate exposed children from those who are also direct victims of abuse, allowing one to determine the unique impact on children of exposure separate from direct abuse. A number of authors have produced partial reviews of this growing body of literature and its limitations (see Edleson, 1999a; Fantuzzo & Lindquist, 1989; Fantuzzo & Mohr, 1999; Holtzworth-Munroe, Smutzler, & Sandin, 1997; Jaffe & Sudermann, 1995; Kashani, Daniel, Dandoy, & Holcomb, 1992; Margolin, 1998; Peled & Davis, 1995; Rossman, 2001). Overall, studies reveal that some children exposed to adult domestic violence exhibit more difficulties than those not so exposed. These difficulties can be grouped into two major categories: (1) behavioral and emotional functioning, and (2) cognitive functioning and attitudes. These two areas, and the degree to which these problems extend into young adulthood, are reviewed below.

Behavioral and Emotional Problems

Several studies report that children exposed to domestic violence exhibit more aggressive and antisocial behaviors (often called "externalized" behaviors), as well as fearful and inhibited behaviors ("internalized" behaviors), when compared to nonexposed children (Fantuzzo et al., 1991; Hughes, 1988; Hughes, Parkinson, & Vargo, 1989). Exposed children also show lower social competence than other children (Adamson & Thompson, 1998; Fantuzzo et al., 1991) and higher than average anxiety, depression, trauma symptoms, and temperament problems than children not exposed to violence at home (Hughes, 1988; Maker, Kemmelmeier, & Peterson, 1998; Sternberg et al., 1993).

A common question is whether exposed children go on to commit more violence when compared to groups of other children. Social learning theory suggests that children who witness violence might also learn to use it. There is some support for this hypothesis. For example, Singer, Miller, Guo, Slovak, and Frierson (1998) found that recent exposure to violence in the home was a significant factor in predicting a child's violent behavior outside the home.

Cognitive and Attitudinal Problems

A number of studies measure the association between cognitive development problems and exposure to adult domestic violence. While academic abilities were not found to differ between exposed and other children in one study (Mathias, Mertin, & Murray, 1995), another found increased violence exposure associated with lower cognitive functioning (Rossman, 1998). One consequence of witnessing violence may be the attitudes a child develops concerning the use of violence and conflict resolution. Spaccarelli, Coatsworth, and Bowden's (1995) findings support this association by showing that, among a sample of adolescent boys incarcerated for violent crimes, those exposed to family violence believed more than others that "acting aggressively enhances one's reputation or self-image," and holding this belief significantly predicted violent offending. It appears that boys and girls may also differ in what they learn from these experiences. Carlson (1991) found that boys exposed to domestic violence were on average significantly more likely to approve of violence than were girls who had also witnessed it.

Longer-Term Problems

A third category of associated problems cuts across the other two and provides evidence of longer-term development issues for exposed children. For example, Silvern et al.'s (1995) study of undergraduate students found that exposure to violence as a child was associated with adult reports of depression, trauma-related symptoms, and low self-esteem among women, versus only trauma-related symptoms among men. Violence exposure appears to be independent of the problems accounted for by the existence of parental alcohol abuse and divorce. In the same vein, Henning, Leitenberg, Coffey, Turner, and Bennett (1996) found that adult women who witnessed domestic violence as children experienced greater distress and lower social adjustment when compared to nonexposed adults. These findings persisted even after accounting for the effects of witnessing parental verbal conflict, being abused as a child, and level of reported parental caring.

Children's Varying Experiences

Most readers will be convinced by the foregoing studies that children exposed to domestic violence must all show evidence of greater problems than other children. In fact, the picture is not so clear. These studies compared groups of children who were either exposed or not exposed to domestic violence. The results reported are group trends and may or may not indicate an individual child's experience. In fact, the available research reveals a great deal of variability in children's experiences and the impact of those experiences on a child.

Graham-Bermann (2001) points out that many children exposed to domestic violence show no greater problems than children not so exposed. At least two recent studies support this claim. For example, a study of children living in a shelter and recently exposed to domestic violence found great variability in problem symptoms (Hughes & Luke, 1998). Over half the children in the study were classified as either "doing well" ($n = 15$) or "hanging in there" ($n = 21$). Children "hanging in there" exhibited average levels of problems and low self-esteem, and some mild anxiety symptoms. The remaining children in the study did show problems: nine showed "high behavior problems," another nine "high general distress," and four were labeled "depressed kids." In a more recent study, Grych, Jouriles, Swank, McDonald, and Norwood (2000) found that, of 229 shelter resident children, 71 exhibited no problems, another 41 showed only mild distress symptoms, 47 exhibited externalized problems, and 70 were classified as multiproblem. Finally, Sullivan, Nguyen, Allen, Bybee, and Juras (2000a) studied 80 7- to 11-year-old children of 80 mothers with a recent history of domestic violence. The children reported they were happy with themselves (83%), liked their physical appearance (83%), and felt they often do the right thing (73%). Their mothers also reported their children to be relatively healthy on a behavioral checklist. It appears that at least half the children in these studies were surviving the experience with few or no problems evident.

How do we explain these findings? On the one hand, it may be that our measures are just not sensitive enough to observe the entire range of harm done to these children through exposure to violence. It may also be that we have not followed children long enough to determine the true impact of violence exposure. On the other hand, it is also highly likely that children's experiences vary greatly in a number of ways:

- The level of violence in each family.
- The degree to which each child is exposed to that violence.
- Other stressors to which a child may be exposed.
- The harm it produces for each child.
- How resilient a child and his or her environment is to violence exposure.

These factors require a closer examination.

Level of Violence in Families

First, the level of domestic violence varies greatly across families. For example, the 1985 National Family Violence Survey (Straus & Gelles, 1990) reveals that an estimated 8.7 million American couples (16.1%) annually experience at least one incident of domestic violence. It also found, however, that 3.4 million American couples (6.3%) annually experience violence that is more severe and has a higher risk of causing injury. Straus and Gelles (1990) reviewed dozens of other studies that show similar variation among families. In general, variation in the types, frequency, and severity of violent events in a family is a well-documented phenomenon. In addition, as will be shown below, there is great variation in the degree to which both adult domestic violence and child maltreatment co-occur in families.

Level of Child Exposure to Violence

Second, it is very likely that children's exposure to violence at home and what meaning they attach to it varies greatly (Peled, 1998). For example, Edleson, Mbilinyi, Beeman, and Hagemeister (2003) found that 45% of the 114 mothers they anonymously interviewed reported their children came into the room where abuse was occurring at least occasionally, while 18% reported that their children frequently came into the room, and 23% reported their children never came into the room. Hughes (1988) found that all 40 child witnesses she studied were "either present in the same room and saw the fighting or were in an adjacent room and heard the physical conflict." In another study, even when one or both parents reported that their children had not seen the violence, approximately 21% of their children reported seeing it (O'Brien, John, Margolin, & Erel, 1994). These studies offer just some examples of the great variance among children's experiences.

Exposure to Other Stressors

Children's experiences vary not just in their exposure to adult domestic violence. Children likely have varying risk and protective factors present in their lives (Hughes, Graham-Bermann, & Gruber, 2001; Masten & Coatsworth, 1995). Risk factors that co-occur with domestic violence might include parental substance abuse, presence of weapons in the home, both maternal and male caregiver mental health issues, and other neglect. Parental substance abuse and domestic violence co-occur in many families, although the level of this overlap varies based on class and the sample studied (Bennett, 1998). The presence of firearms is also associated with an increase in domestic homicides (Saltzman, Mercy, O'Carroll, Rosenberg, & Rhodes, 1992; Kellermann et al., 1993). Parental or caregiver mental health issues may also result from or be a source of domestic violence (Campbell, Kub, & Rose, 1996; Golding, 1999; Goodman, Koss, & Russo, 1993). These and other factors may combine with domestic violence in some families to create greater risk of neglect or abuse. In fact, some child protection workers argue that families in which domestic violence occurs are often substantiated for child neglect only after other risk factors such as substance abuse by parents or the presence of weapons are found to exist.

Risk of Harm

The risk of harm resulting from exposure may also vary from child to child, and must be examined in terms of (1) the degree to which a child is involved in violent events and (2) the documented level of child maltreatment and emotional harm. Children's immediate responses to violent situations may increase the risk for their own well-being. Their responses vary from becoming actively involved in the conflict, to distracting themselves and their parents, or to distancing themselves (Margolin, 1998). Their responses also vary by gender and age. For example, Garcia O'Hearn, Margolin, and John (1997) studied 110 families and found that parents whose conflict was often characterized by physical violence reported that their boys were significantly more likely than other boys in the study to respond to conflict by leaving the room or appearing sad or frightened. This difference was not significant for girls.

Other studies find a wider variety of responses by children. For example, Peled's (1998) qualitative study of 14 preadolescent children exposed to domestic violence reveals children use two primary strategies when adult domestic violence occurs: distancing oneself from the event or intervening directly in it. Some children who distanced themselves use televisions or loud music to distract themselves, while others "willed away" their feelings and thoughts about the events. Those children who got involved in events took sides in arguments, protected their abused mothers by "jumping in the middle of it," or called the police. On one level, many of these strategies may be seen as successful coping, while on another level some may also be seen as efforts by the child to dissociate and reflect the impact of earlier trauma.

Children of different ages also show some variation in their responses to violent conflict at home. In one of the earliest studies on this subject, Cummings, Zahn-Waxler, and Radke-Yarrow (1981) reported that children between the ages of 1 and 2½ years respond to angry conflict, including physical attacks, with negative emotions such as crying, and efforts to become actively involved in the conflicts. In a later study, Cummings, Pellegrini, Notarius, and Cummings (1989) found that as children age, they increasingly observe the conflict, express concern, seek social support, and intervene to protect or comfort their mothers. This effect is greater among children whose parents were engaged in physical conflict when compared to others, and among boys when compared to girls. In a more recent study, Adamson and Thompson (1998) examined children's response strategies. Children from homes in which there is violence were nine times more likely to use verbal or physical aggression to intervene in parental conflict than were children from violence-free homes (27% vs. 3%). Finally, Edleson et al.'s (2003) study found that 52% of 114 mothers reported that their children yelled from another room during abusive events at least occasionally, and 24% reported their children frequently yelled from another room. Twenty-one percent of the mothers reported their children called someone else for help during the abuse at least occasionally, and 6% reported they did so frequently. Twenty-three percent of the mothers reported that their children became physically involved during an abusive incident involving the mother at least occasionally, 8% reported that their children physically intervened frequently, but almost 45% reported that their children never intervened physically.

Overall, these studies show children respond in a variety of ways to real and simulated violent conflict between their parents. It is not surprising, then, that the emotional and physical harm that children exhibit may also vary, and that the risk created by such responses will vary accordingly. The data on risk of physical harm to children also indicate great variability. A number of reviews currently exist on the co-occurrence of documented child maltreatment in families where adult domestic violence is also occurring. Over 30 studies of the link between these two forms of violence show a 40% median co-occurrence of child maltreatment and adult domestic violence in families studied (Appel & Holden, 1998) and a range of co-occurrence from as low as 6.5% and as high as 97%, depending on the samples studied (Edleson, 1999b).

Resilience

There is a growing research literature on children's resilience in the face of trauma (see, for example, Garmezy, 1974; Werner & Smith, 1992; Garmezy & Masten, 1994). The surprise in these research findings is that many children exposed to trauma show no greater problems than nonexposed peers, leading Masten (2001) to label such widespread resilience as "ordinary magic."

The resilience literature suggests that as assets in a child's environment increase, the problems he or she experiences may actually decrease (Masten & Reed, 2002). The harm children experience may be moderated by a number of factors, including how a child interprets or copes with the violence (see Hughes, Graham-Bermann, & Gruber, 2001). Sternberg et al. (1993) suggest that "perhaps the experience of observing spouse abuse affects children by a less direct route than physical abuse, with cognitive mechanisms playing a greater role in shaping the effects of observing violence."

A number of other factors also affect the degree to which a child is harmed by violence. For example, whether or not a child is also a direct victim of abuse seems associated with the degree of harm experienced. Hughes et al. (1989) found that children who were both abused and exposed exhibited the most severe problem behaviors, a witness-only group showed moderate problem symptoms, and a comparison no-exposure group the least. This same pattern appears in a series of other comparison group and correlational studies (see Carlson, 1991; Hughes, 1988; O'Keefe, 1994; and Sternberg et al., 1993). Children seem to agree; for example, in one study, the children indicated that being abused or both abused and a witness had a greater negative impact based on their self-ratings of problems than witnessing adult domestic violence alone (McClosky, Figueredo, & Koss, 1995).

Gender appears to be another factor that affects the types of problems experienced. In general, boys exhibit more frequent problems and ones that are categorized as externally oriented, such as hostility and aggression. Girls generally show evidence of more internally oriented problems, such as depression and somatic complaints (Carlson, 1991; Stagg, Wills, & Howell, 1989). There are also findings that dissent from this general trend by showing that girls, especially as they get older, may exhibit more aggressive behaviors (for example, Spaccarelli, Sandler, & Roosa, 1994). Children of different ages appear to exhibit differing responses associated with witnessing violence, with children in preschool exhibiting more problems than other age groups (Hughes, 1988). Children also exhibit fewer problems the longer the period of time since their last exposure to a violent event. For example, Wolfe, Zak, Wilson, and Jaffe (1986) found more social problems among children residing in shelters than among children who had at one time in the past resided in a shelter. The immediate turmoil of recent violence may temporarily escalate child problems observed in a shelter setting.

Finally, a number of authors discuss a child's relationship with adults in the home as a key factor moderating the impact of violence. There is some conjecture that a mother's poor mental health negatively affects a child's experience of violence, but the data are conflicting. Levendosky and Graham-Bermann (1998) found that the children of mothers exhibiting stress showed more problem behaviors themselves. McClosky et al. (1995) found, however, that mothers' poor mental health did not affect a child's response to violence in the home.

One apparent problem in the few studies that examine parent–child relationship factors is an overreliance on measures of the mother–child relationship, while little data exist about father–child relationships in families where the father or other adult male is violent (Sternberg, 1997). Holden and Ritchie (1991) found that while both maternal stress and reports of the fathers' irritability accounted for the variation in problems of children exposed to domestic violence, only maternal stress accounted for significant variation in comparison with nonexposed children's problems. In a somewhat similar vein, Sullivan, Juras, Bybee, Nguyen, and Allen (2000b) found that the relationship of an abusive male to the child directly affected the child's well-being, without being mediated by the mother's level of mental health. In particular, stepfathers in their sample seemed to be more emotionally abusive to the children, and the children feared them more, when compared to biological fathers and unrelated male partners in the home.

Unfortunately, we do not yet clearly understand what helps some children survive violence exposure better than others. It may be that the "ordinary magic" of protective factors in everyday life play a major role in how children experience and cope with exposure to violence at home (see Edleson & Gewirtz, 2002).

LEGISLATIVE RESPONSES
TO CHILDHOOD EXPOSURE

It is clear from the literature reviewed above that children exposed to adult domestic violence are sometimes at risk for developing a series of behavioral, emotional, cognitive, and attitudinal problems that may persist into adulthood. It is also clear that children from homes where adult domestic violence occurs are at a greater risk for being abused themselves. Yet, within the groups of exposed children, many do not exhibit problems and do not themselves become victims of child abuse. We do not yet know which children are safe and recover quickly once in a safe environment and which may develop short- or long-term problems. So where do these conclusions lead us? Across North America, one response has been passage of new legislation in both the criminal and civil law arenas (Weithorn, 2001). These changes affect the way in which the criminal justice agencies, child protection systems, and domestic violence programs respond to families in which children are exposed to adult domestic violence.

New Laws on Childhood Exposure

As discussed in detail in Chapters 11 and 12, at least 16 states, Puerto Rico, and one Canadian province have revised their criminal and civil laws to specifically address the needs of children exposed to adult domestic violence (NCJFCJ, 2000). For example, a Utah law (Utah Code Ann. §76-5-109.1) passed in July 1997 makes the commission of adult domestic violence two or more times in the presence of a child a separate criminal offense from the assault itself. In California, the presence of children may bring enhanced criminal penalties in adult assault cases, and in Oregon a misdemeanor assault may be elevated to a felony if minors were present (Cal. Penal Code §1170.76, Or. Rev. Stat. §163.160).

Expanding the Definition of Maltreatment

Another approach is to expand the definition of child maltreatment to include children who have witnessed domestic violence. In 1999 the Minnesota State Legislature expanded the definition of child neglect to include exposure to adult domestic violence as a specific type of neglect

(Minn. State Ann. §626.556, see Minnesota Department of Human Services, 1999). The change in Minnesota acknowledges what has long been believed to be the practice in many county child protection agencies across the state—accepting certain reports of children's exposure to adult domestic violence as child neglect, and taking them into the child protection system as "failure to protect" cases. For instance, in a study of one Minnesota county's child protection system prior to the 1999 changes in definition, 19% of child maltreatment reporters were aware of adult domestic violence in the home, and 36.4% of the child maltreatment reports investigated included some evidence of similar violence (Edleson & Beeman, 1999). In the same study, cases with domestic violence present were more likely to be rated as high-risk (50.7% vs. 33.3%) by child protection investigators and opened for service (45.6% vs. 24.4%) when compared to those without evidence of domestic violence. Interestingly, more than three-quarters (76.3%) of the cases that were cited as "failure to protect" contained indications of adult domestic violence (Edleson & Beeman, 1999).

Minnesota is not alone in including such families in its neglect caseloads. Exposure to domestic violence is commonly included in published definitions of child neglect (see English, 1998; Kalichman, 1999). The National Clearinghouse on Child Abuse and Neglect Information suggests that operational definitions of child neglect across the United States should include "spouse abuse in the child's presence" (NCCANCH, 2002, p. 2), and this definition is found internationally as well. For example, most Canadian provinces already include exposure to domestic violence in their definitions of child maltreatment (Weithorn, 2001). The Australian province of New South Wales passed the Children and Young Persons (Care and Protection) Act of 1998 that defines reportable forms of child risk as a child or young person "living in a household where there have been incidents of domestic violence and, as a consequence, the child or young person is at risk of serious physical or psychological harm" (Australasian Legal Information Institute, 2001). After Minnesota's Reporting Act was initially changed, most counties in Minnesota experienced a 50% to 100% increase in child protection reports that involved exposure to adult domestic violence (see Minnesota Association of Community Social Service Administrators, 2000). County child welfare agency administrators estimate that this seemingly simple and unfunded change in the law created the need for over $30 million in expanded services to newly identified children and families. The experience was so overwhelming for child protection agencies that the Minnesota Legislature repealed the change in April 2000. The legislature never reinstituted the change due to insufficient funding for children's services.

Defining Exposure as Maltreatment under the Law

There is a national consensus that children at risk for harm should receive the attention of our social institutions. Ideally, a child protection agency's interventions should lead to enhanced child safety and family strengths when there is a reported concern about a child. Such systems should also be part of a rich network of community-based institutions offering additional support to families. In reality, our child protection systems are given so few public resources that they most often only respond to the cases of children at the greatest risk. This leaves most children—including those exposed to domestic violence—and their families the subject of screening and investigation by child protection systems, but without the provision of many subsequent services. Nationally, estimates are that 40%–60% of families in which maltreatment is substantiated receive no further services (English, 1998).

There are several possible responses to this situation. Many advocate full investigations of all families where children have been exposed to violence, regardless of cost. Others take a more pragmatic and resource-sensitive position, standing against expanding the number and types of children referred to an already overburdened child protection system. And still others seek to minimize involvement with the child protection system because of its perceived harsh treatment of some families. These positions are likely to harden as several lawsuits against child protection agencies move forward. In New York City, lawyers for several battered mothers filed suit against the city for removing the mothers' children from their custody for failing to protect the children from witnessing domestic violence committed against the mothers. The judge ruled that the city's child protection system violated parents and children's constitutional right to due process by removing children from mothers solely because the mothers were victims of domestic violence (Family Violence Prevention Fund, 2001).

A NEW WAY TO DEFINE CHILDHOOD EXPOSURE AS MALTREATMENT

Positions that argue for defining childhood exposure as maltreatment or against doing so all have some merit but often leave many confused about where to stand on these issues. Does one stand for child safety and demand more societal resources? Or does one recognize the practical reality of both resources and current practice and avoid unnecessarily involving families in systems that ultimately may not now or may never have the resources to provide them with adequate help? There is another way to look at this situation that draws on the strengths of each of these positions. This common ground can be found in three major tenets:

1. Childhood exposure to adult domestic violence should not automatically be defined as maltreatment under the law.
2. *Many* children and their families should not be referred for forensic child protection investigations and interventions that carry the possibility of legal action against the parents. Rather, they should be offered voluntary, community-based assessments and services.
3. *Some* children exposed to adult domestic violence are at great risk for harm, and should be referred to the child protection system for assessment and intervention with their families.

These statements form the basis for a reasoned approach to this issue that is both safety- and resource-sensitive. Each is described in more detail below.

1. *Exposure should not be defined as maltreatment per se.* As the data presented earlier in this chapter clearly document, there is great variability in children's experiences with adult domestic violence. Studies of families experiencing adult domestic violence show that anywhere from 3% to 92% of the children in these homes are also maltreated, depending on the families studied (Edleson, 1999a). Large numbers of children studied show no greater problems than their peers who are not so exposed, but other children exhibit multiple problems at a level thought to require clinical intervention. These data argue strongly that we should not automatically define a child's exposure to adult domestic violence as a form of child maltreatment.

One could argue that most forms of child maltreatment vary greatly, but we still include them in mandatory reporting rules so that a full child protection screening and investigation can be conducted. I would argue, however, that we already exclude other forms of child exposure from such screening and investigation. These include corporal punishment, some degrees of substance abuse by caregivers, and exposure to both second-hand smoke and violent media, to name a few. For instance, not all physical hitting of children is defined as child abuse. Straus (1994) aptly describes how spanking and other forms of corporal punishment of children are not, in most cases, defined as child maltreatment in our culture. There is increasing documentation of children's exposure to community and school-based violence (Freeman, Hartmut, & Poznanski, 1993; Garbarino, Kostelny, & Dubrow, 1991; Osofsky,

Wewers, Hann, & Fick, 1993), yet the focus of social intervention is on primary prevention in communities (Office of Juvenile Justice and Delinquency Prevention, 2000). It is also true that substance abuse by a caregiver is not defined as maltreatment unless it is shown to present a significant risk to a child, for example, in the case of prenatal exposure (Chasnoff & Lowder, 1999).

Efforts have been made in recent years to focus child protective services more narrowly on the most severe cases, allowing other types of family problems to be better handled through voluntary assessments and family support services (see Waldfogel, 1998). In most cases, children exposed to adult domestic violence should fall into this "other" category.

2. *Many exposed children and their families may benefit from voluntary, community-based services instead of the traditional child protection services.* The data presented in this chapter also suggest that many exposed children and their families might benefit from early screening and intervention focused on strengthening existing personal, social, and economic resources, and on stopping the perpetrators' violent behavior. Many battered women's shelters and community-based domestic violence programs have long provided services to children who have witnessed violence (see Peled & Davis, 1995). Several other community-based programs provide trauma treatment and social support for exposed children and their families. For example, the Child Witness to Violence Project (CWVP) at Boston Medical Center was founded in 1992 with the goal of providing therapy services for children who had witnessed various forms of violence in the community. The CWVP now provides services for children to heal from the trauma of violence exposure and for parents to help their children, works closely with domestic violence and other community agencies to help families find safety, and offers intensive training for a variety of professionals (see Groves, Roberts, & Weinreb, 2000).

Voluntary, community-based assessment and intervention services for exposed children and their families are woefully underdeveloped, even though they have a long history in battered women's programs. Attention to the development, expansion and evaluation of these services should be a top priority for all communities.

3. *Some exposed children and their families should be referred to Child Protection Services.* Understanding the varying risk to children also leads to acknowledging that some exposed children should be referred to child protection services. There is no doubt that some children in families where domestic violence occurs are in imminent danger of harm, and action may need to be taken quickly. Some children are also exposed to a combination of several risk factors such as pa-

rental substance abuse or neglect that requires child protection involvement. One way to differentiate those requiring a report to child
protective services would be to develop a series of criteria and/or
screening instruments that, based on available or new data, indicate
heightened risk for children. For example, these criteria could include
domestic violence occurring with other risk factors such as: the presence of weapons; the proximity or actions of the child in violent situations; the presence of an alcohol- or drug-abusing caregiver; and/or the
history of the abusive partner's including repeated or severe violence in
the home. At this point, the field is too new to have determined these
criteria, but it is an area with which both child protection systems and
community-based agencies need a great deal of assistance in defining
and refining.

   Magen, Conroy, and Del Tufo (2000) published one of the few specific studies describing a comprehensive domestic violence assessment in
child welfare prevention settings. Their experience in New York City
was that identification can be enhanced, was appreciated by clients, and
that new domestic violence services were added as a result of the new assessments. Greater expertise must be developed within child protection
agencies for those families that are assessed to require further intervention. This may take the form of developing "differential" responses to
families that include more supportive and voluntary service opportunities in addition to traditional child protection responses (see Waldfogel,
1998; Minnesota Department of Human Services, 2000). In addition,
child protection systems must adopt new strategies and develop both internal expertise and collaborative relationships with domestic violence
agencies in working with families where adult domestic violence exists
(see Beeman & Edleson, 2000; Findlater & Kelly, 1999; National Council of Juvenile and Family Court Judges, 1998, 1999; Whitney & Davis,
1999). These internal responses should include safety planning and support for abused mothers and children as well as expanded intervention
with perpetrators of adult violence.

SUMMARY AND CONCLUSIONS

This chapter examined both current knowledge about the risks to children exposed to adult domestic violence and the concerns that some may
be jumping to the conclusion that all children exposed to domestic violence should be redefined under the law as maltreated children. There is
no need to redefine child neglect to be inclusive of all children exposed
to domestic violence. The children most harmed by exposure to domestic violence may already be reported to child protection agencies under

existing laws. Empirical and practice-based criteria for deciding whether or not a child is at a heightened risk of harm are badly needed in this field. These criteria, once established, must be developed into effective and psychometrically tested screening and assessment instruments for use in the field. In addition, there is also a dire need to develop greater expertise within child protection agencies, collaboration with domestic violence programs, and alternative forms of voluntary, community-based services for exposed children and their families, including specialized parenting and batterer intervention programs. Child protection agencies will be seen as the first intervention of choice until these alternatives exist in sufficient numbers across the country.

REFERENCES

Adamson, J. L., & Thompson, R. A. (1998). Coping with interparental verbal conflict by children exposed to spouse abuse and children from nonviolent homes. *Journal of Family Violence, 13*, 213–232.

Appel, A. E., & Holden, G. W. (1998). The co-occurrence of spouse and physical child abuse: A review and appraisal. *Journal of Family Psychology, 12*, 578–599.

Australasian Legal Information Institute. (2001). *New South Wales Consolidated Acts: Children and Young Persons (Care and Protection) Act 1998 B Section 23.* Retrieved February 20, 2001, from: *http://www.austlii.edu.au/legis/nsw/consol_act/.*

Beeman, S. K., & Edleson, J. L. (2000). Collaborating on family safety: Challenges for children's and women's advocates. *Journal of Aggression, Maltreatment and Trauma, 3*(1), 345–358. (Copublished in R. Geffner & P. G. Jaffe, *Children exposed to family violence: Intervention, prevention, and policy implications.* Binghamton, NY: Haworth Press.)

Bennett, L. W. (1998). *Substance abuse and woman abuse by male partners.* Harrisburg, PA: VAWnet B National Electronic Network on Violence Against Women—*http://www.vawnet.org*

California Penal Code §1170.76.

Campbell, J., Kub, J. E., & Rose, L. (1996). Depression in battered women. *Journal of the American Medical Women's Association, 51*, 106–112.

Carlson, B. E. (1991). Outcomes of physical abuse and observation of marital violence among adolescents in placement. *Journal of Interpersonal Violence, 6*, 526–534.

Chasnoff, I. J., & Lowder, L. A. (1999). Prenatal alcohol and drug use and risk for child maltreatment. In H. Dubowitz (Ed.), *Neglected children: Research, practice, and policy* (pp. 132–155). Thousand Oaks, CA: Sage.

Cummings, E. M., Zahn-Waxler, C., & Radke-Yarrow, M. (1981). Young children's responses to expressions of anger and affection by others in the family. *Child Development, 52*, 1274–1282.

Cummings, J. S., Pellegrini, D. S., Notarius, C. I., & Cummings, E. M. (1989). Children's responses to angry adult behavior as a function of marital distress and history of interparental hostility. *Child Development, 60,* 1035–1043.

Edleson, J. L. (1999a). The overlap between child maltreatment and woman battering. *Violence Against Women, 5*(2), 134–154.

Edleson, J. L. (1999b). Children's witnessing of adult domestic violence. *Journal of Interpersonal Violence, 14*(8), 839–870.

Edleson, J. L., & Beeman, S. B. (1999). *Final report: Responding to the co-occurrence of child maltreatment and adult domestic violence in Hennepin County.* St. Paul, MN: University of Minnesota—*http://www.mincava.umn.edu/ link.*

Edleson, J. L., & Gewirtz, A. (2002, May 16–17). *Young children's exposure to adult domestic violence: The case for early childhood research and intervention.* Paper presented at "Early Childhood, Domestic Violence, and Poverty: Taking the Next Steps to Help Young Children and Their Families," Children's Defense Fund, Washington, DC.

Edleson, J. L., Mbilinyi, L. F., Beeman, S. K., & Hagemeister, A. K. (2003). How children are involved in adult domestic violence: Results from a four city telephone survey. *Journal of Interpersonal Violence, 18*(1), 18–32.

English, D. J. (1998). The extent and consequences of child maltreatment. *The Future of Children, 8,* 39–53.

Family Violence Prevention Fund. (2001, December 21). Draft injunction favors battered women in New York City lawsuit. *Speaking Up, 7*(23), 1–4.

Fantuzzo, J. W., DePaola, L. M., Lambert, L., Martino, T., Anderson, G., & Sutton, S. (1991). Effects of interparental violence on the psychological adjustment and competencies of young children. *Journal of Consulting and Clinical Psychology, 59,* 258–265.

Fantuzzo, J. W., & Lindquist, C. U. (1989). The effects of observing conjugal violence on children: A review and analysis of research methodology. *Journal of Family Violence, 4,* 77–94.

Fantuzzo, J. W., & Mohr, W. K. (1999). Prevalence and effects of child exposure to domestic violence. *The Future of Children, 9,* 21–32.

Findlater, J. E., & Kelly, S. (1999). Reframing child safety in Michigan: Building collaboration among domestic violence, family preservation, and child protection services. *Child Maltreatment, 4*(2), 167–174.

Freeman, L. N., Hartmut, M., & Poznanski, E. O. (1993). Violent events reported by normal urban school-aged children: Characteristics and depression correlates. *Journal of the American Academy of Child and Adolescent Psychiatry, 32,* 419–423.

Garbarino, J., Kostelny, K., & Dubrow, N. (1991). What children can tell us about living in danger. *American Psychologist, 46,* 376–383.

Garcia O'Hearn, H., Margolin, G., & John, R. S. (1997). Mothers' and fathers' reports of children's reactions to naturalistic marital conflict. *Journal of the American Academy of Child and Adolescent Psychiatry, 36,* 1366–1373.

Garmezy, N. (1974). The study of competence in children at risk for severe psychopathology. In E. J. Anthony & C. Koupernik (Eds.), *The child in his family: Vol. 3. Children at psychiatric risk* (pp. 77–97). New York: Wiley.

Garmezy, N., & Masten, A. (1994). Chronic adversities. In M. Rutter, E. Taylor, & L. Hersov (Eds.), *Child and adolescent psychiatry: Modern approaches.* Oxford, UK: Blackwell Scientific.

Golding, J. M. (1999). Intimate partner violence as a risk factor for mental disorders: A meta-analysis. *Journal of Family Violence, 14,* 99–132.

Goodman, L. A., Koss, M. P., & Russo, N. F. (1993). Violence against women: Physical and mental health effects. Part I: Research findings. *Applied and Preventive Psychology, 2,* 79–89.

Graham-Bermann, S. A. (2001). Designing intervention evaluations for children exposed to domestic violence: Applications of research and theory. In S. A. Graham-Bermann & J. L. Edleson (Eds.), *Domestic violence in the lives of children: The future of research, intervention, and social policy* (pp. 237–267). Washington, DC: American Psychological Association.

Groves, B. M., Roberts, E., & Weinreb, M. (2000). *Shelter from the storm: Clinical intervention with children affected by domestic violence.* Boston: Boston Medical Center.

Grych, J. H., Jouriles, E. N., Swank, P. R., McDonald, R., & Norwood, W. D. (2000). Patterns of adjustment among children of battered women. *Journal of Consulting and Clinical Psychology, 68,* 84–94.

Henning, K., Leitenberg, H., Coffey, P., Turner, T., & Bennett, R. T. (1996). Long-term psychological and social impact of witnessing physical conflict between parents. *Journal of Interpersonal Violence, 11,* 35–51.

Holden, G. W., & Ritchie, K. L. (1991). Linking extreme marital discord, child rearing, and child behavior problems: Evidence from battered women. *Child Development, 62,* 311–327.

Holtzworth-Munroe, A., Smutzler, N., & Sandin, B. (1997). A brief review of the research on husband violence. Part II: The psychological effects of husband violence on battered women and their children. *Aggression and Violent Behavior, 2,* 179–213.

Hughes, H. M. (1988). Psychological and behavioral correlates of family violence in child witness and victims. *American Journal of Orthopsychiatry, 58,* 77–90.

Hughes, H. M., Graham-Bermann, S. A., & Gruber, G. (2001). Resilience in children exposed to domestic violence. In S. A. Graham-Bermann & J. L. Edleson (Eds.), *Domestic violence in the lives of children: The future of research, intervention, and social policy* (pp. 67–90). Washington, DC: American Psychological Association.

Hughes, H. M., & Luke, D. A. (1998). Heterogeneity in adjustment among children of battered women. In G. W. Holden, R. Geffner, & E. N. Jouriles (Eds.), *Children exposed to marital violence* (pp. 185–221). Washington, DC: American Psychological Association.

Hughes, H. M., Parkinson, D., & Vargo, M. (1989). Witnessing spouse abuse and experiencing physical abuse: A "double whammy"? *Journal of Family Violence, 4,* 197–209.

Jaffe, P. G., & Suderman, M. (1995). Child witnesses of woman abuse: Research and community responses. In S. M. Stith & M. A. Straus (Eds.), *Understanding partner violence* (pp. 213–222). Minneapolis, MN: National Council on Family Relations.

Jouriles, E. N., McDonald, R., Norwood, W. D., & Ezell, E. (2001). Issues and controversies in documenting the prevalence of children's exposure to domestic violence. In S. A. Graham-Bermann & J. L. Edelson, (Eds.), *Domestic violence in the lives of children* (pp. 11–34). Washington, DC: American Psychological Association.

Kalichman, S. C. (1999). *Mandated reporting of suspected child abuse* (2nd ed.). Washington, DC: American Psychological Association.

Kashani, J. H., Daniel, A. E., Dandoy, A. C., & Holcomb, W. R. (1992). Family violence: Impact on children. *Journal of the American Academy of Child and Adolescent Psychiatry, 31,* 181–189.

Kellermann, A. L., Rivara, F. P., Rushforth, N. B., Banton, J. G., Reay, D. T., Francisco, J. T., Locci, A. B., Prodzinski, J., Hackman, B. B., & Somes, G. (1993). Gun ownership as a risk factor for homicide in the home. *New England Journal of Medicine, 329,* 1084–1091.

Levendosky, A. A., & Graham-Bermann, S. A. (1998). The moderating effects of parenting stress on children's adjustment in woman-abusing families. *Journal of Interpersonal Violence, 13,* 383–397.

Magen, R. H., Conroy, K., & Del Tufo, A. (2000). Domestic violence in child welfare preventative services: Results from an intake screening questionnaire. *Children and Youth Services Review, 22,* 251–274.

Maker, A. H., Kemmelmeier, M., & Peterson, C. (1998). Long-term psychological consequences in women of witnessing parental physical conflict and experiencing abuse in childhood. *Journal of Interpersonal Violence, 13,* 574–589.

Margolin, G. (1998). Effects of witnessing violence on children. In P. K. Trickett & C. J. Schellenbach (Eds.), *Violence against children in the family and the community* (pp. 57–101). Washington, DC: American Psychological Association.

Masten, A. S. (2001). Ordinary magic: Resilience processes in development. *American Psychologist, 56,* 227–238.

Masten, A. S., & Coastworth, D. (1998). The development of competence in favorable and unfavorable environments. *American Psychologist, 53,* 205–220.

Masten, A. S., & Reed, M. (2002). Resilience in development. In C. R. Snyder & S. J. Lopez, (Eds.), *Handbook of positive psychology.* Oxford, UK: Oxford University Press.

Mathias, J. L., Mertin, P., & Murray, A. (1995). The psychological functioning of children from backgrounds of domestic violence. *Australian Psychologist, 30,* 47–56.

McClosky, L. A., Figueredo, A. J., & Koss, M. P. (1995). The effects of systemic family violence on children's mental health. *Child Development, 66,* 1239–1261.

Minnesota Association of Community Social Service Administrators. (2000). *Co-occurring spouse abuse and child abuse: Domestic violence fiscal note—January 2000.* St. Paul, MN: Author.

Minnesota Department of Human Services. (1999). *Bulletin #99-68-15: Laws related to domestic violence involving children, including 1999 amendments to neglect definition in Maltreatment of Minors Act.* St. Paul, MN: Author.

Minnesota Department of Human Services. (2000). *Bulletin #00-68-4: DHS issues guidance on Alternative Response to reports of child maltreatment.* St. Paul, MN: Author.

Minnesota State Ann. §626.556.

National Clearinghouse on Child Abuse and Neglect Information. (2002, February). *What is child maltreatment?* Retrieved October 2, 2003, from: *http://www.calib.com/nccanch/pubs/factsheets/childmal.cfm.*

National Council of Juvenile and Family Court Judges. (1998). *Family violence: Emerging programs for battered mothers and their children.* Reno, NV: Author.

National Council of Juvenile and Family Court Judges. (1999). *Effective intervention in domestic violence and child maltreatment: Guidelines for policy and practice.* Reno, NV: Author.

National Council of Juvenile and Family Court Judges. (2000, September). *Criminal and civil state legislation pertaining to domestic violence committed in the presence of a child.* Reno, NV: Author.

O'Brien, M., John, R. S., Margolin, G., & Erel, O. (1994). Reliability and diagnostic efficacy of parents' reports regarding children's exposure to marital aggression. *Violence and Victims, 9,* 45–62.

Office of Juvenile Justice and Delinquency Prevention. (2000). *Safe from the start: Taking action on children exposed to violence.* Washington, DC: Author.

O'Keefe, M. (1994). Linking marital violence, mother–child/father–child aggression, and child behavior problems. *Journal of Family Violence, 9,* 63–78.

O'Leary, K. D., Slep, A. M. S., & O'Leary, S. G. (2000). Co-occurrence of partner and parent aggression: Research and treatment implications. *Behavior Therapy, 31,* 631–648.

Oregon Revised Statute §163.160.

Osofsky, J. D., Wewers, S., Hann, D. M., & Fick, A. C. (1993). Chronic community violence: What is happening to our children? *Psychiatry, 56,* 36–45.

Peled, E. (1998). The experience of living with violence for preadolescent witnesses of woman abuse. *Youth and Society, 29,* 395–430.

Peled, E., & Davis, D. (1995). *Group work with children of battered women.* Thousand Oaks, CA: Sage.

Rossman, B. B. (1998). Descartes's Error and posttraumatic stress disorder: Cognition and emotion in children who are exposed to parental violence. In G. W. Holden, R. Geffner, & E. N. Jouriles (Eds.), *Children exposed to marital violence* (pp. 223–256). Washington, D.C.: American Psychological Association.

Rossman, B. B. R. (2001). Long-term effects of exposure to adult domestic violence. In S. A. Graham-Bermann & J. L. Edleson (Eds.), *Domestic violence in the lives of children: The future of research, intervention, and social policy* (pp. 35–66). Washington, DC: American Psychological Association.

Saltzman, L. E., Mercy, J. A., O'Carroll, P. W., Rosenberg, M. L., & Rhodes, P. H. (1992). Weapon involvement and injury outcomes in family and intimate assaults. *Journal of the American Medical Association, 267,* 3043–3047.

Silvern, L., Karyl, J., Waelde, L., Hodges, W. F., Starek, J., Heidt, E., & Min, Kyung (1995). Retrospective reports of parental partner abuse: Relationships to depression, trauma symptoms and self-esteem among college students. *Journal of Family Violence, 10,* 177–202.

Singer, M. I., Miller, D. B., Guo, S., Slovak, K., & Frierson, T. (1998). *The mental health consequences of children's exposure to violence.* Cleveland, OH: Cayahoga County Community Mental Health Research Institute, Mandel School of Applied Social Sciences, Case Western Reserve University.

Spaccarelli, S., Coatsworth, J. D., & Bowden, B. S. (1995). Exposure to serious family violence among incarcerated boys: Its association with violent offending and potential mediating variables. *Violence and Victims, 10,* 163–182.

Spaccarelli, S., Sandler, I. N., & Roosa, M. (1994). History of spouse violence against mother: Correlated risks and unique effects in child mental health. *Journal of Family Violence, 9,* 79–98.

Stagg, V., Wills, G. D., & Howell, M. (1989). Psychopathology in early childhood witnesses of family violence. *Topics in Early Childhood Special Education, 9,* 73–87.

Sternberg, K. J. (1997). Fathers, the missing parents in research on family violence. In M. E. Lamb (Ed.), *The role of the father in child development* (3rd ed., pp. 284–309). New York: Wiley.

Sternberg, K. J., Lamb, M. E., Greenbaum, C., Cicchetti, D., Dawud, S., Cortes, R. M., Krispin, O., & Lorey, F. (1993). Effects of domestic violence on children's behavior problems and depression. *Developmental Psychology, 29,* 44–52.

Straus, M. A. (1994). *Beating the devil out of them: Corporal punishment in American families.* New York: Lexington Books.

Straus, M. A., & Gelles, R. J. (1990). *Physical violence in American families.* New Brunswick, NJ: Transaction.

Sullivan, C. M., Juras, J., Bybee, D., Nguyen, H., & Allen, N. (2000b). How children's adjustment is affected by their relationships to their mothers' abusers. *Journal of Interpersonal Violence, 15,* 587–602.

Sullivan, C. M., Nguyen, H., Allen, N., Bybee, D., & Juras, J. (2000a). Beyond searching for deficits: Evidence that physically and emotionally abused women are nurturing parents. *Journal of Emotional Abuse, 2,* 51–71.

Utah Code Ann. §76-5-109.1.

Waldfogel, J. (1998). Rethinking the paradigm for child protection. *The Future of Children, 8*(1), 104–119.

Weithorn, L. A. (2001). Protecting children from exposure to domestic violence: The use and abuse of child maltreatment statutes. *Hastings Law Journal, 53(1),* 1–156.

Werner, E. E., & Smith, R. S. (1992). *Overcoming the odds: High-risk children from birth to adulthood.* Ithaca, NY: Cornell University Press.

Whitney, P., & Davis, L. (1999). Child abuse and domestic violence in Massachusetts: Can practice be integrated in a public child welfare setting? *Child Maltreatment, 4*(2), 158–166.

Wolfe, D. A., Zak, L., Wilson, S., & Jaffe, P. (1986). Child witnesses to violence between parents: Critical issues in behavioral and social adjustment. *Journal of Abnormal Child Psychology, 14,* 95–104.

3

Young Children Exposed to Adult Domestic Violence

Incidence, Assessment, and Intervention

B. B. ROBBIE ROSSMAN, JACQUELINE G. REA,
SANDRA A. GRAHAM-BERMANN, and PERRY M. BUTTERFIELD

Exposure to repetitive adult domestic violence may be just as traumatizing for many young children as personal experience of maltreatment (Scheeringa & Gaensbauer, 2000). In fact, Scheeringa and Zeanah (1995) found that children under the age of 4 years who witnessed a threat to their caregivers showed more posttraumatic stress disorder (PTSD) hyperarousal symptoms as well as more new fears and aggression than did children who did not. In addition, children who witnessed traumatic events happening to someone else showed more hyperarousal symptoms than did children who directly experienced the event. It seems likely that exposure to domestic violence may be accompanied by similar behavioral difficulties and posttraumatic dysregulation in the stress response system. These types of findings highlight the importance of attending to the well-being of young children exposed to domestic violence.

The goals of this chapter are to: (1) review what is known about the incidence of exposure of children to adult domestic violence; (2) suggest methods for assessing the developmental and trauma status of young exposed children ages 0–6 years; and (3) review programs that currently assist abused mothers and their young children. Because the age range from 0 to 6 years is broad in terms of children's developmental needs and tasks, we discuss all issues by incidence for children ages 0–3 years, and then for preschool children (4–6 years).

INCIDENCE OF EXPOSURE
FOR YOUNG CHILDREN

Domestic violence and children's exposure to it contribute significantly to health, psychiatric, and productivity problems in our country. An estimated 1.8–4 million women are victims of domestic abuse in the United States each year (Novello, 1992), and as many as 10 million children are exposed to domestic violence (Straus, 1991). Nearly 50% of abusive husbands batter their pregnant wives, resulting in four times the risk of low birth weight and a higher than expected level of birth defects (Chiles, 1988; U.S. Senate Hearings, 1990). Shahinfar (1997), working with children 3.5–4.5 years of age, found that 78% had been exposed to violence, with 41.9% exposed to violence in the home. Fantuzzo, Boruch, Beriana, Atkins, and Marcus (1997) report that households with domestic violence in five major U.S. cities had a significantly higher proportion of children under 5 years of age (40–49%) than would be expected based on census data, and that children in this age range were disproportionately exposed to multiple incidents of domestic violence. An estimated 37–63% of exposed children are also abused and/or neglected (Aron & Olsen, 1997). See Chapter 2 for a discussion of the impact of exposure to violence on children.

ASSESSMENT METHODS
FOR CHILDREN 0–3 YEARS OF AGE

Possibly more than at any other age, assessments of infants and toddlers require the gathering of information from multiple sources and about multiple aspects of a child's behavior and life (Gilliam & Mayes, 2000; Zero to Three, 1994). However, this comment and much of the information below can also be applied to preschoolers. This information gathering includes learning about the child's developmental milestones and history, including:

- Pregnancy and delivery information
- The child–caregiver(s) relationship patterns
- The child's temperament
- The child's affective, language, motor, cognitive, and sensory reactions and capabilities
- Information about the parents as individuals
- Patterns of family functioning in his or her culture and community

This also includes gaining information from caregivers, structured tests or tasks, medical records, and observations of the child and caregiver–child interactions. When called for, such information can be used to make a formal Axis I diagnosis of a disorder using the *Diagnostic Classification of Mental Health and Developmental Disorders of Infancy and Early Childhood* (DC:0–3; Zero to Three, 1994). Community agencies may not need to diagnose, but will want to do as thorough a screening as possible for potential referral for additional evaluation or treatment.

A special issue arises for exposed children regarding the process used for giving feedback to abused mothers. While any parent of a young child is sensitive to concerns voiced by professionals, abused mothers may be especially vulnerable and highly sensitive to news of developmental delays or difficulties of their young child. They are parenting under a great deal of stress (Levendosky & Graham-Bermann, 1998), and often do not have social or financial resources to help them cope with such information. As a result, the feedback needs to be structured as part of a treatment plan. The impact of the information needs to be considered, and child and maternal strengths as well as community and coping resources should be highlighted (Zeanah, 1998).

When screening, it is most helpful if the developmental assessment device used actually provides information based on parent report, direct observation, and some standardized tasks. In particular, observations of predominant affective tone, engagement, use of others, and reactions to transitions are useful, because how a child carries out a task may indicate how the child approaches learning new skills (Gilliam & Mayes, 2000). Observation of mother–child interactions can be helpful as well. For example, is a child able to be calmed by his or her mother or follow the mother's instructions? What is the most common affective tone of interactions (e.g., positive, anxious, angry)? While beyond the scope of this chapter, there are domains (e.g., parental emotional availability and child emotion regulation, Sameroff & Emde, 1989) and systems for parent–child relationship assessment (Zeanah, Larrieu, Heller, & Valliere, 2000). There are also special systems for organizing and communicating the direct observations of the child. One of these systems is called the Infant and Toddler Mental Status Exam (ITMSE; American Academy of Child and Adolescent Psychiatry, 1997; Benham, 2000), for children 0–5 years of age.

Finally, there are helpful formal assessment devices that provide developmental norms. It should be noted that all assessment devices require adequate training if the administration is to be valid. There are three useful types of tests, depending on the amount of time available and the goal of the assessment. Multidomain developmental tests are typically based on Gesell's (1940) original model in which child development unfolds simultaneously in distinct but related domains. These tests require assessment in five areas: personal–social; motor; communication; cognition; and adaptive functioning. The Bayley Scales of Infant Development–II (BSID-II; Bayley, 1993) provide a good multidomain assessment for children 0–42 months old, but are often too time-consuming for screening purposes, taking up to an hour for children over 1.5 years. Other tests focus on cognition as a predictor of later performance. The Cattell Infant Intelligence Scale (Cattell, 1960) provides a good example of this approach, assessing general intelligence up to 30 months.

Screening tests probably provide the most feasible option for use in community agencies. They are intended to be brief, but cover several domains and relate well to more comprehensive instruments such as the BSID-II. Gilliam and Mayes (2000) provide a list of current screening devices. One example is the Denver Developmental Screening Test–II (DDST-II; Frankenberg et al., 1990). The DDST-II is frequently used for screening children 0–6 years old because it typically takes only 15–20 minutes to administer and includes a parent report, observation of the child, and standard assessment items. The test assesses four domains based on the different inputs: personal–social; fine-motor-adaptive; gross motor; and language. The results place children in overall categories of normal, questionable, abnormal, or untestable. The DDST-II shows reasonable agreement with more comprehensive devices such as the BSID-II (Frankenberg, Goldstein, & Camp, 1991). However, there are two concerns about the DDST-II: the norming sample, while large and inclusive of disadvantaged children seen in neighborhood health clinics, was entirely from the state of Colorado; and, there is evidence that the test overidentifies children as having problems (Glascoe & Byrne, 1993).

Another screening test that has many of the same features as the DDST-II, including a norming sample from one location (southwestern Ontario), is the Diagnostic Inventory for Screening Children–4 (DISC-4; Amdur, Mainland, & Parker, 1996). This device can be used for children ages 0–5 years to provide assessment in fine and gross motor skills, expressive and receptive language, auditory and visual attention and memory, and personal–social and adaptive functioning.

One other commonly used questionnaire is the Child Behavior Checklist/2–3 (CBCL/2–3; Achenbach, 1992). This checklist has a form for parents and a similar Caregiver–Teacher report form for children ages 2–5. These checklists assess problem behaviors in the areas of: anxiety/depression; withdrawal; sleep; somatic problems; aggressive problems; and destructive behavior. Other screening devices are available, but few cover the 0–3 age range and assess multiple domains based on the recommended three sources of information (i.e., direct observation, parent report, and structured test items).

A final critical area to assess for young children is posttraumatic symptomatology. None of the procedures mentioned above accomplishes this. The only documented procedure currently available for children ages 0–3 years is provided by Scheeringa, Zeanah, Drell, & Larrieu (1995), for children up to 48 months of age. This procedure involves a parent interview regarding the incidence of the typical DSM-IV PTSD symptoms for his or her child in addition to some alternative symptoms (e.g., the development of new fears or aggression), which are specific to young children's expression of trauma. For children 2 years and older, a trauma play observation segment can also be included. This procedure provides the scoring for both DSM-IV criteria and alternative PTSD criteria for young children, which agree well with the DSM-IV diagnoses. The alternative criteria appear to yield a larger number of diagnoses than the traditional criteria in existing research (Rossman et al., 2001; Scheeringa et al., 1995). However, this may be entirely suitable, because the point of the new procedure is to provide a more developmentally appropriate assessment.

In summary, it is important to assess exposed children ages 0–3 years to inform referral and treatment needs. We strongly recommend a short history taking, general developmental screening device, and at least the parent interview for child PTSD as part of an initial screening procedure. Early identification is important for early intervention and for hopefully avoiding the cumulative cascade of problems and child distress that may unfold for exposed children when difficulties are not noted.

INTERVENTION PROGRAMS
FOR CHILDREN AGES 0–3 YEARS

Intervention may be critical for exposed young children because research now shows that the problems, symptoms, or delays of exposed older children may not automatically remediate. In addition, research shows that abused mothers and children benefit from being out of the violent home, but that further benefits are realized from receiving services, especially home-based services.

Evidence is emerging from the child abuse literature that traumatic experiences occurring or beginning during the first 3 years of life may be especially noteworthy (Ogawa, Sroufe, Weinfield, Carlson, & Egeland, 1997; Warren, Huston, Egeland, & Sroufe, 1997). Thus, Kaufman and Henrich (2000) suggest broad and comprehensive interventions for traumatized children. These interventions should be responsive to children's current psychological symptoms of all types; developmental deficits; problems in the parenting environment, such as spousal violence; problems in the children's living environments, such as poverty; and trauma-specific reactions. The interventions discussed below are responsive to one or more of these areas of risk, as are the treatment recommendations of Gaensbauer (1996).

Interventions involving home-based services could provide a useful addition to many agency programs for abused mothers. Two components of these programs are especially important: (1) helping abused mothers obtain needed living resources and providing personal and parenting support for them; and (2) including guided interactions so that mothers and young children can share positive affect in their relationship, so mothers can come to understand their children's behavior and learn how to avoid power struggles.

There are at least two examples of successful home-based programs for at-risk mothers with young children (Lieberman, Silverman, & Pawl, 2000, for disadvantaged mothers; Olds, Kitzman, Cole, & Robinson, 1997, for teen mothers). The program described by Olds et al. (1997) is known as Home Visitation 2000 (HV2000). This program was designed as a preventative intervention for high-risk mothers—often teen mothers—where there were no identified client-specific problems, but living circumstances of poverty and other factors placed them and their babies at risk. The goals of the program include:

- Attending to the use of informal social support for adaptive behavior change
- Identifying and promoting the use of needed community services

- Working in a culturally sensitive way with the help of ethnically diverse home visitors and supervisors
- Working from a strengths- or accomplishments-based approach, or getting the person to perform parts of a desired behavior to set up the expectation of efficacy
- Building anticipatory coping skills
- The home visitor modeling desired behaviors in the context of a warm therapeutic relationship with the mother
- The home visitor forming a warm therapeutic alliance with the mother or parents
- The home visitor understanding with the parent the parent's own care-receiving history and its connection to the parent's current role as caregiver
- Promoting sensitive and responsive caregiving by helping mothers learn to read child cues, elicit desired child behaviors, and enhance positive emotional and behavioral interaction between the parent and child

The program has outcome goals at several levels, including the physical and psychological health of the mother and baby and the integration of the mother into a helping community of family, friends, community, and culture. This program demonstrated success in health, child development, and maternal parenting and self-sufficiency outcomes with three sets of random trials with large groups of Anglo, African American, and Hispanic families.

The second approach, the Infant–Parent Psychotherapy Program (Lieberman et al., 2000), has as its identified target a troubled parent–child relationship, and the mutually constructed meanings in this relationship. This program is designed both for immediate treatment and ultimate prevention purposes. The program is based on the therapist's efforts to understand how the parent's current and past relationship experiences influence the parent's perceptions, feelings, and behaviors toward the child. In addition, the baby's contribution to influencing the interaction in terms of his or her physical or temperamental characteristics that hold meaning for the parents is considered. Because one component of this program focuses on the mutual construction of meaning in the parent–child pair, how the child participates in this process should also be addressed. For example, are the child's cues accepted and incorporated, or are the parent's meanings imposed? Are the child's behaviors so anxiously responded to that they dictate the relationship?

The infant's behavior, its developmental meaning, and the needed parental response become what Lieberman et al. (2000) call one "port of entry" into the therapeutic process. What the child can display about his or her understandings of self and relationship to others provides another.

Valuable developmental and relational learning is provided when the parent learns to understand how the child interprets the parent's behavior, and when the child has that understanding validated and perhaps corrected by the parent. This program has had success with disadvantaged and ethnically diverse populations, as well as in pilot work with abused mothers and preschoolers where the abuser has left the home.

In practice, both of these approaches have similar elements, including:

- Facilitating the positive interaction of the parent–child pair
- Using the therapeutic alliance and a support- and strength-based approach rather than evaluation-based approach to helping
- Providing developmental information
- Understanding and helping the parent understand how his or her own past and current relationship experiences have shaped his or her self-understanding and his or her understanding of the child and their relationship
- Providing concrete assistance for living
- Being ethnically sensitive and having demonstrated usefulness with ethnically diverse populations

Differences between the programs arise in the broader, more ecological, parent and child, and family and community orientation of HV2000, as compared with the focus on a troubled parent–child pair of the Infant–Parent Psychotherapy approach. It is possible that in different situations one or the other approach could be more useful.

Another option for abused mothers of young children are the longer-term shelter-sponsored apartment unit residences where some services are offered. These longer-term options are very limited, because most shelters cannot afford them and, where available, the number of families that can be accommodated is small. In addition, an informal survey of three Denver area shelters which do have all three types of services suggests that 75–85% of crisis shelter families with young children leave the shelter without continuing services, about 5% use the shelter weekly out-client services, and about 5% can be accommodated in the longer-term programs. Thus, there is clear need for additional service options.

A PILOT STUDY OF A HOME-BASED INTERVENTION PROGRAM

Research suggests (Posada, Liu, & Johnson, in press) that domestic violence may make it difficult for mothers and children to form secure emotional relationships. Given these findings, our lab conducted a small pilot study of a home-based intervention for 20 battered mothers with children ages 1–3 years, most of whom were living in low-income single-parent housing. We used components similar to those common to the above approaches, and were also assisted by Sullivan, Campbell, Angelique, Eby, and Davidson's (1994) and Jouriles et al.'s (2001) home visitor programs, which were primarily directed toward battered mothers with older children. One particularly important feature we borrowed from Jouriles et al.'s (2001) program was the provision of both a designated therapist (i.e., a master's-level clinical graduate student or therapist) and a child specialist [BA-level psychology major] in our home visitor teams). The child specialist worked to assist the therapist but, more importantly, carried out activities with older siblings, typically ranging from ages 4–7 years. These activities were designed to carry out the major theme for each visit (e.g., recognition of emotional cues). This was a very helpful addition, because most families had one to three older siblings who could benefit, and it left the therapist with uninterrupted time to work with the mother and toddler. In fact, these activities were so welcomed by the siblings that they began to invite their friends to join them. Unfortunately, we needed to restrict this because it created too much chaos in the home.

Our intervention was a brief multicomponent intervention program that considered contextual, maternal, child, and intervention influences, as did the HV2000 model (Olds et al., 1997). The major program components were derived from the home visitation programs discussed above, especially from Jouriles et al. (2001) and Sullivan and Bybee (1999): social advocacy, self-efficacy, parenting and the mother–child relationship, and attention to contextual adversity and support. The parenting and mother–child attachment component was provided by a curriculum adapted from the Partners in Parenting Education (PIPE) parent training program (Butterfield, 1996), which is a standard component of HV2000 and has been used successfully by early Head Start and child abuse programs, and school-based classes for teenage mothers. Intervention components included:

- How to listen to an infant/toddler and understand his or her cues and needs (Listen, Listen, Listen)
- Issues regarding attachment and emotion regulation (Love Is Layers of Sharing)
- The use of play and positive emotions to motivate and scaffold learning and language (Playing Is Learning)

Materials and worksheets for each topic are written for parents with limited reading skills and incorporate instruction as well as crafts, games, and interactive tasks. The self-efficacy components target increasing the mothers' sense of mastery through learning effective parenting practices and honing solution-focused problem-solving skills (O'Brien & Baca, 1997). These skills can then be used to decrease stressors and obtain needed community and social resources, jobs, and occupational/educational training to facilitate self-sufficiency.

Unfortunately, given the brief nature of this pilot intervention study, with an average of seven home visits over 3–5 months, we were not able to demonstrate treatment effects for the objective measures (e.g., BSDI-II scores), once the children's initial scores on these measures were controlled. Our preintervention measures indicated trauma symptoms and problems with emotion regulation and motor quality by up to half of the children. Mothers who continued with the program reported that the program was very useful, that they felt increased positive interactions with their toddler, and that it provided them with greater understanding of their toddler's behavior and how to manage it. They also provided good, PIPE-based "advice" to another "hypothetical" mother in about 90% of responses during postprogram interviews, demonstrating their mastery of the parenting materials.

ASSESSMENT METHODS FOR PRESCHOOLERS

Similar to work with children 0–3 years old, assessment for preschoolers benefits greatly from the use of multiple informants and methods that provide information from multiple developmental domains. Preschoolers have greater language fluency and therefore can tell us more in words. However, because their words may not reflect all of their understandings, their play may be very informative. Several broader, though not complete, developmental batteries are available for administration to 2½- to 7-year-old children: The Wechsler Preschool and Primary Scale of Intelligence, Third Edition (WPPSI-III; Wechsler, 2002); the McCarthy Scales of Intelligence (McCarthy, 1972); and, starting at age 6, the Wechsler Intelligence Scale for Children, Fourth Edition (WISC-IV; Wechsler, 2003). These scales provide information in the following areas: general cognitive ability; verbal comprehension; perceptual organization/nonverbal reasoning; and short-term memory. Thus, these types of instruments provide broader assessment of general abilities.

There are also screening devices that extend upward to 5 or 6 years, as noted by Gilliam and Mayes (2000). The DDST-II and Diagnostic Inventory for Screening Children–4 were mentioned earlier. Two other multiple source devices that are appropriate to age 6 are the Developmental Indicators for the Assessment of Learning—Revised (DIAL-R; Mardell-Czudnowski & Goldenberg, 1990) and the Early Screening Profile (ESP; Harrison, 1990). The DIAL-R was normed on a large and representative sample, has acceptable psychometric properties, and provides assessment of the following domains: motor; academic or preacademic skills; expressive and receptive language; and behavior. The ESP has norms from a representative sample, good psychometric properties, and assesses five areas: expressive and receptive language; articulation; cognition; motor skills; and adaptive and personal–social behaviors. While based only on parent report, the Vineland (Sparrow, Balla, & Cicchetti, 1984) and Adaptive Behavior Scales for Children (Mercer & Lewis, 1978) provide more extensive information about adaptive functioning if that is an issue. Problem behaviors and social competence can be assessed more specifically using Child Behavior Checklist instruments, as noted earlier. There is a Caregiver–Teacher Report Form for Ages 2–5, a Teacher Report Form for ages 6–11, and a parent report form. The Child Behavior Checklist/4–18 (Achenbach, 1991) can be used for 4- to 18-year-olds.

A problem arises in trying to assess trauma symptoms for preschoolers, because they fall in the gap of coverage between younger and older children. Scheeringa et al.'s (1995) parent interview and child trauma play procedure can be used up to 4 years of age and possibly further. The Child PTSD Reaction Index (Pynoos et al., 1987; Pynoos, Nader, & March, 1991) was modified with pictures for administration with children as young as 5 years (Rossman, Bingham, & Emde, 1997), and the elementary age version of this could be used with 6-year-olds. The Trauma Symptom Checklist for Children (Briere, 1995) elementary age version could also possibly be used with 6-year-olds. A potential concern regarding the use of the last three scales is that the children need to respond to questions containing words they may or may not understand. Reading the questions with young children is advised. However, these scales have the advantage that their instructions can be modified so that one is asking the child about symptoms resulting from parental violence incidents. This does not guarantee that their symptom report is specific to those incidents, but it is a start. In addition, Richters and Martinez (1993) developed a scale for school-age children that assesses symptoms in relation to community violence exposure. Some combination of child report, observation, and parent report may be useful for assessing trauma symptoms for the in-between preschool age group. Again, we recommend that some form of developmental and trauma screening be used for exposed preschoolers.

INTERVENTION PROGRAMS FOR PRESCHOOLERS

Many shelters and communities offer education, support, or intervention programs for children and battered women. Until recently, there has been little empirical evidence based on systematic research that these interventions help the children (National Research Council, 1998). Because a disproportionate number of young children witness and are at risk for violence exposure, and because many communities and shelters are financially strapped in providing for the multiple needs of families in distress, the information obtained from the systematic evaluation of programs is essential to making the best use of these scarce resources. Rigorous intervention studies are just beginning to be reported and show promising, if preliminary, results in improving the social and emotional functioning of some young children who experience family violence in their lives (Graham-Bermann, 2001).

Intervention programs for young children are most commonly offered in shelters and in community settings. Young exposed children often present with fairly specific problems, as mentioned above, yet many interventions address a broad range of problems. Most often, programs seek to (1) enhance the child's coping, (2) build social skills, and (3) reduce the negative effects of violence exposure. Not every program includes the child's parent in the intervention.

In 1982, Honore Hughes created and implemented one of the first treatment groups for children of battered women—the Program for Sheltered Children (Hughes, 1982). This original program served both shelter preschool and school-age children and their mothers. The program aimed to foster parenting skills, build children's self-esteem, reduce anxiety, and improve coping behavior, along with altering attitudes toward family violence. This program relied in part on cognitive-behavioral therapy, where children received additional information that helped them to reframe their particular scripts related to the use of violent behavior (Kendall, 1985). Preliminary evaluation with a sample of 12 children and mothers suggests that levels of anxiety were reduced for both following this intervention (Hughes, 1982; Hughes & Barad, 1983). However, a larger sample, a control group, and follow-up assessment would help to demonstrate the stability of the reported change.

A 10-session weekly program named The Storybook Club by Tutty and Wagar (1994) was designed to teach problem solving, conflict resolution, and safety skills to 5- to 7-year-old children of battered women, and was evaluated. Cox (1995) studied this program for 13 children ages 5–7 from low-income families and found that children experienced a significant reduction in anxiety following the intervention. Taking a social learning approach, this program supposes that some young children learn to be either aggressive or withdrawn following exposure to adult domestic violence (Patterson, 1982). Thus, they are at risk for developing roles as either victims or perpetrators of violence (Huesmann, Eron, Loefkowitz, & Walder, 1984). Using a developmentally appropriate approach for working with young children, this program relies on stories that are both read to children and acted out. The evaluation is limited because the sample is small and there is no follow-up evaluation.

Another program that relies on a social learning theory paradigm is Project SUPPORT, created by Jouriles and colleagues (Jouriles et al., 2001). This program is specifically targeted to children rated high in conduct problems following exposure to domestic violence. This multifaceted program seeks to provide children with alternative models of problem solving to develop and then reinforce nonviolent conflict resolution strategies. Thus, each child works with a mentor who gives support and serves as a role model for the mother. In addition, mothers participate in parenting support aimed at helping them to develop resources, including their strengths as parents. Trained therapists provide the parenting support for the mother. The program was evaluated with 36 children and mothers who were assessed at three time points, including an 8-month postintervention follow-up (Jouriles et al., 2001). Families were randomly assigned to intervention and comparison groups. Results show that conduct problems in the child were reduced and parenting skill enhanced for the intervention group as compared to the nontreatment group.

The Groupwork with Child Witnesses to Domestic Violence program by Peled and Edleson (1992) was evaluated to assess whether children exposed to adult domestic violence could change attitudes about violence, disclose their emotional responses to the violence, and learn alternative strategies for coping with violence in a supportive atmosphere. Children ages 4–12 were accepted into the program if they separated comfortably from their mothers, had an adequate attention span, and interacted socially in the small group setting. The evaluation study (Peled & Edleson, 1992; Peled & Davis, 1995) used qualitative methods to interview mothers of 30 children following the last intervention session. Results indicate that children were able to discuss the violence and disclose their emotional reactions.

The Preschool Kids' Club program is a 10-week intervention with young children exposed to violence in the family (Graham-Bermann & Follett, 2000). The intervention targets 3- to 6-year-old children's knowledge about family violence, their attitudes and beliefs about families and family violence, their fears and worries, and their social behavior in the small-group setting. One of the goals of this program is to reduce children's anxiety as well as to reduce conduct problems. An evaluation of 181 children of a school-age version of The Kids' Club program shows that significant change from baseline was found in cognition (children's increased knowledge about violence, safety planning), social interactions (improved social skills, emotion regulation), and in emotional/behavioral domains (reduced anxiety as well as behavioral symptoms) (Graham-Bermann, Lynch, & Halabu, 2002). When both the mother and the child received intervention, the effects in all areas were greater than for the children-only intervention group or for the comparison group (Graham-Bermann, 2001).

While the need for early intervention with this population of children is clear, it is also evident that any effective intervention for this age group will include support for mothers. The 10-week parenting program that accompanies The Kids' Club program empowers the mother to identify her own and her child's needs when coping with stress related to adult domestic violence, to develop a safety plan, and to reconnect with sources of instrumental and social support (Graham-Bermann & Levendosky, 1994). This program was developed and tested with three groups of preschool-age children exposed to recent severe domestic violence. The advocacy and support components of the mothers' groups have proven effective in other shelter and community programs for battered women (e.g., Sullivan & Bybee, 1999). This program is described in more detail in Chapter 5.

SUMMARY AND CONCLUSIONS

The foregoing discussion and review suggest that children ages 0–6 years who have been exposed to domestic violence are at risk for troubled developmental paths. This implies that further research is needed to determine more about the developmental and trauma status of these young children and their mothers, and to use some form of assessment to understand more about how each child is doing. Research suggests that levels of symptoms among older children living in shelters may vary and require different types and levels of intervention (e.g., Hughes, Graham-Bermann, & Gruber, 2001). We do not know this about very young children or children in the community, but should undertake such investigations.

Interventions that assist young exposed children with accomplishing developmental tasks and reducing trauma may often be needed, and there are models available, as reviewed above. However, further rigorous research is also needed to evaluate program outcomes and which children are best treated by which types of programs. Program fidelity, lack of a comparison group, small samples, what outcomes to measure when, and how to deal with the lack of a preexposure baseline for child functioning are all problems that need to be addressed. Finally, the nature of the developmental tasks taking place rapidly during this time and the critical role of the mother–child relationship in this process underscore the importance of nurturing that relationship and the mothers' well-being.

REFERENCES

Achenbach, T. M. (1991). *Manual for the Child Behavior Checklist/4-18 and 1991 Profile*. Burlington, VT: University of Vermont Department of Psychiatry.

Achenbach, T. M. (1992). *Manual for the Child Behavior Checklist/2-3 and 1992 Profile*. Burlington, VT: University of Vermont Department of Psychiatry.

Amdur, J. R., Mainland, M. K., & Parker, K. C. H. (1996). *Diagnostic Inventory for Screening Children (DISC) manual (4th ed.)*. Kitchener, Ontario: Kitchener-Waterloo Hospital.

American Academy of Child and Adolescent Psychiatry. (1997). Practice parameters for the psychiatric assessment of infants and toddlers (0–36 months). *Journal of the American Academy of Child and Adolescent Psychiatry, 36,* 215–365.

Aron, L. Y., & Olson, K. K. (1997, Summer). Efforts by child welfare agencies to address domestic violence. *Public Welfare,* 4–13.

Bayley, N. (1993). *Bayley Scales of Infant Development* (2nd ed.). San Antonio, TX: Psychological Corporation.

Benham, A. L. (2000). The observation and assessment of young children including use of the infant–toddler mental status exam. In C.H. Zeanah, Jr. (Ed.), *Handbook of infant mental health* (2nd ed., pp. 249–265). New York: Guilford Press.

Briere, J. (1995). *Trauma Symptom Checklist for Children*. Odessa, FL: Psychological Assessment Resources, Inc.

Butterfield, P. M. (1996, August–September). The partners in parenting education program: A new option in parent education. *Bulletin of Zero to Three: National Center for Infants, Toddlers, and Families, 17,* 3–10.

Cattell, P. (1960). *Cattell Infant Intelligence Scale*. Cleveland: Psychological Corporation.

Chiles, L. (1988). Report of the National Commission to Prevent Infant Mortality, *Death Before Life: The Tragedy of Infant Mortality* (16).

Cox, G. M. (1995). *Changes in self esteem and anxiety in children in a group program for witnesses of wife assault*. Unpublished master's thesis, School of Social Work, University of Calgary, Calgary, Alberta, Canada.

Fantuzzo, J. W., Boruch, R., Beriana, A., Atkins, M., & Marcus, S. (1997). Domestic violence and children: Prevalence and risk in five major cities. *Journal of the American Academy of Child and Adolescent Psychiatry, 36,* 116–122.

Frankenburg, W. K., Dodds, J., Archer, P., Bresnick, B., Maschka, P., Edelman, N., & Shapiro, H. (1990). *Denver II: Technical manual*. Denver, CO: Denver Developmental Materials.

Frankenburg, W. K., Goldstein, A. D., & Camp, B. W. (1971). The revised Denver Developmental Screening Test: Its accuracy as a screening instrument. *Journal of Pediatrics, 79,* 988–995.

Gaensbauer, T. (1996). Development and therapeutic aspects of treating infants and toddlers who have witnessed violence. In J. D. Osofsky & E. Fenichel (Eds.), *Islands of safety: Assessing and treating young victims of violence* (pp. 15–20). Washington, DC: Zero to Three: National Center for Infants, Toddlers, and Families.

Gesell, A. (1940). *The first five years of life: A guide to the study of the preschool child.* New York: Harper.

Gilliam, W. S., & Mayes, L. C. (2000). Developmental assessment of infants and toddlers. In C. H. Zeanah, Jr. (Ed.), *Handbook of infant mental health* (2nd ed., pp. 236–248). New York: Guilford Press.

Glascoe, F. P., & Byrne, K. E. (1993). The accuracy of three developmental screening tests. *Journal of Early Intervention, 17,* 368–379.

Graham-Bermann, S. A. (2001). Designing intervention evaluations for children exposed to domestic violence: Applications of research and theory. In S. A. Graham-Bermann & J. Edleson (Eds.), *Domestic violence in the lives of children: The future of research, intervention, and social policy* (pp. 237–267). Washington, DC: American Psychological Association.

Graham-Bermann, S. A., & Follett, C. (2000). *The Preschool Kids' Club: A preventive intervention program for children of battered women.* Department of Psychology, University of Michigan.

Graham-Bermann, S. A., & Levendosky, A. A. (1994). *The moms' group: A parenting support and intervention program for battered women who are mothers.* Ann Arbor: University of Michigan.

Graham-Bermann, S. A., Lynch, S., & Halabu, H. (2002). *Testing models of effects of interventions to reduce anxiety, depression and aggression in children of battered women.* Manuscript in preparation.

Harrison, P. L. (1990). *Early Screening Profiles (ESP): Manual.* Circle Pines, MN: American Guidance Service.

Huesmann, L. R., Eron, L. D., Loefkowitz, M. M., & Walder, L. O. (1984). Stability of aggression over time and generations. *Developmental Psychology, 20,* 1120–1134.

Hughes, H. (1982). Brief interventions with children in a battered women's shelter: A model program. *Family Relations, 31,* 495–502.

Hughes, H., & Barad, S. (1983). Psychological functioning of children in a battered women's shelter: A preliminary investigation. *American Journal of Orthopsychiatry, 53*(3), 525–531.

Hughes, H. M., Graham-Bermann, S. A., & Gruber, G. (2001). Resilience in children exposed to domestic violence. In S. A. Graham-Bermann & J. L. Edleson (Eds.), *Domestic violence in the lives of children: The future of research, intervention, and social policy* (pp. 91–110). Washington, DC: American Psychological Association.

Individuals with Disabilities Education Act Amendments of 1986, Pub. L. No. 99–457 §303 (1986).

Jouriles, E. N., McDonald, R., Spiller, L., Norwood, W. D., Swank, P. R., Stephens, N., Ware, H., & Buzy, W. M. (2001). Reducing conduct problems among children of battered women. *Journal of Consulting and Clinical Psychology, 69*(5), 774–785.

Kaufman, J., & Henrich, C. (2000). Exposure to violence and early childhood trauma. In C. H. Zeanah, Jr. (Ed.), *Handbook of infant mental health* (2nd ed., pp. 195–207). New York: Guilford Press.

Kendall, P. C. (1985). Toward a cognitive-behavioral model of child psychopathology and a critique of related interventions. *Journal of Abnormal Child Psychology, 13,* 357–372.

Levendosky, A. A., & Graham-Bermann, S. A. (1998). The moderating effects of parenting stress on children's adjustment in woman-abusing families. *Journal of Interpersonal Violence, 13,* 383–397.

Lieberman, A. F., Silverman, R., & Pawl, J. H. (2000). Infant–parent psychotherapy: Core concepts and current approaches. In C. H. Zeanah, Jr. (Ed.), *Handbook of infant mental health* (2nd ed., pp. 472–484). New York: Guilford Press.

Mardell-Czudnowski, C. D., & Goldenberg, D. (1990). *DIAL-R (Developmental Indicators for the Assessment of Learning-Revised).* Edison, NJ: Childcraft Education.

McCarthy, D. A. (1972). *Manual for the McCarthy Scales of Children's Abilities.* San Antonio, TX: Psychological Corporation.

Mercer, J. R., & Lewis, J. F. (1978). *System of Multicultural Pluralistic Assessment.* San Antonio, TX: Psychological Corporation.

National Research Council, Institute of Medicine. (1998). *Violence in families: Assessing prevention and treatment programs.* Washington, DC: National Academy of Sciences.

Novello, A. C. (1992). *From the Surgeon General. U.S. Public Health Service.* 23 JAMA 267, at 3132.

O'Brien, R. A., & Baca, R. P. (1997). Application of solution-focused interventions to nurse home visitation for pregnant women and parents of young children. *Journal of Community Psychology, 25,* 47–57.

Ogawa, J. R., Sroufe, L. A., Weinfeld, N. S., Carlson, E. A., & Egeland, B. (1997). Development and the fragmented self: Longitudinal study of dissociative symptomatology in a nonclinical sample. *Development and Psychopathology, 9,* 855–879.

Olds, D., Kitzman, H., Cole, R., & Robinson, J. (1997). Theoretical foundations of a program of home visitation for pregnant women and parents of young children. *Journal of Community Psychology, 25,* 9–25.

Patterson, G. R. (1982). *Coercive family processes.* Eugene, OR: Castalia.

Peled, E., & Davis, D. (1995). *Groupwork with children of battered women.* Thousand Oaks, CA: Sage.

Peled, E., & Edleson, J. (1992) Multiple perspectives on groupwork with children of battered women. *Violence and Victims, 7,* 327–346.

Posada, G., Liu, X. D., & Johnson, S. (in press). Specific domains of marital discord and attachment security in preschoolers. In E. Waters, B. Vaughn, G. Posada, & D. Teti (Eds.), *Patterns of secure base behavior: Q-sort perspectives on attachment and caregiving in infancy and childhood.* Hillsdale, NJ: Erlbaum.

Pynoos, R. S., Frederick, C., Nader, K., Arroyo, W., Steinberg, A., Eth, S., Nunez, F., & Fairbanks, L. (1987). Life threat and posttraumatic stress in school-age children. *Archives of General Psychiatry, 44,* 1057–1063.

Pynoos, R. S., Nader, K., & March, J. (1991). Childhood post-traumatic stress disorder. In J. Weiner (Ed.), *The textbook of child and adolescent psychiatry* (pp. 955–984). Washington, DC: American Psychiatric Press.

Richters, J., & Martinez, P. (1993). The NIMH community violence project: I. Children as victims of and witnesses to violence. *Psychiatry, 56,* 7–21.

Rossman, B. B. R., Bingham, R. D., & Emde, R. N. (1997). Symptomatology and adaptive functioning for children exposed to normative stressors, dog attack, and parental violence. *Journal of the American Academy of Child and Adolescent Psychiatry, 36,* 1–9.

Rossman, B. B. R., Glicken, R., Guest, K., Mikow, L., Milliden, E., & Rea, J. (2001, June). *Toddlers exposed to intimate partner violence.* Paper presented as part of the symposium "Evaluating the social and emotional adjustment of young children exposed to family violence," at the International Conference on Children Exposed to Domestic Violence, "Our Children, Our Future: A Call to Action," London, Ontario, Canada.

Sameroff, A. J., & Emde, R. N. (Eds.). (1989). *Relationship disturbances in early childhood: A developmental approach.* New York: Basic Books.

Scheeringa, M. S., & Gaensbauer, T. J. (2000). Posttraumatic stress disorder. In C. H. Zeanah, Jr. (Ed.), *Handbook of infant mental health* (2nd ed., pp. 369–381). New York: Guilford Press.

Scheeringa, M. S., & Zeanah, C. H. (1995). Symptom expression and trauma variables in children under 48 months of age. *Infant Mental Health Journal, 16,* 259–270.

Scheeringa, M. S., Zeanah, C. H., Drell, M. J., & Larrieu, J. A. (1995). Two approaches to the diagnosis of posttraumatic stress disorder in infancy and early childhood. *Journal of the American Academy of Child and Adolescent Psychiatry, 34,* 191–200.

Shahinfar, A. (1997, April). *Patterns of violence exposure and symptomatology: The effect of variations in context of exposure on preschool children's behavior.* Paper presented at the meeting of the Society for Research in Child Development, Washington, DC.

Sparrow, S. S., Balla, D. A., & Cicchetti, D. V. (1984). *Vineland Adaptive Behavior Scales.* Circle Pines, MN: American Guidance Service.

Straus, M. A. (1991). *Children as witnesses to marital violence: A risk factor for life-long problems among a nationally representative sample of American men and women.* Paper presented at the Ross Roundtable on "Children and Violence," Washington, DC.

Sullivan, C. M., & Bybee, D. L. (1999). Reducing violence using community-based advocacy for women with abusive partners. *Journal of Consulting and Clinical Psychology, 67,* 43–53.

Sullivan, C. M., Campbell, R., Angelique, H., Eby, K. K., & Davidson, W. S. (1994). An advocacy intervention program for women with abusive partners: Six-month follow-up. *American Journal of Community Psychology, 22,* 101–122.

Tutty, L. M., & Wagar, J. (1994). The evolution of a group for young children who have witnessed family violence, *Social Work with Groups, 17*(1/2), 89–104.

U.S. Senate, Committee on the Judiciary, Hearings on Women and Violence. (1990). *Ten Facts About Violence against Women* (at 78, August 29 and December 11).

Warren, L. S., Huston, L., Egeland, B., & Sroufe, L. A. (1997). Child and adolescent anxiety disorders and early attachment. *Journal of the American Academy of Child and Adolescent Psychiatry, 36,* 637–644.

Wechsler, D. (2002). *Manual for the Wechsler Preschool and Primary Scale of Intelligence* (3rd ed.). San Antonio, TX: Psychological Corporation.

Wechsler, D. (2003). *Manual for the WISC-IV Wechsler Intelligence Scale for Children* (4th ed.). New York: Psychological Corporation, Harcourt Brace Jovanovich.

Zeanah, C. H. (1998). Reflections on the strengths perspective. *Signal, 6,* 11–12.

Zeanah, C. H., Jr., Larrieu, J. A., Heller, S. S., & Valliere, J. (2000). Infant–parent relationship assessment. In C. H. Zeanah, Jr. (Ed.), *Handbook of infant mental health* (2nd ed., pp. 222–235). New York: Guilford Press.

Zero to Three. (1994). *Diagnostic classification of mental health and developmental disorders of infancy and early childhood.* Washington, DC: Zero to Three: National Center for Infants, Toddlers, and Families.

4

Group Intervention with Abusive Male Adolescents

DIANE L. DAVIS

In the past decade there has been increased attention and research on the issue of children's exposure to domestic violence, as well as the development of policy and legislation aimed at stopping domestic violence and protecting adult victims and their children, some who are also victims of direct abuse (Wolfe & Jaffe, 2001). Wolfe and Jaffe (2001) note a deficit of intervention and prevention services available to assist families where domestic violence is present, as well as research on these programs. Likewise, there is a need for research on prevention and intervention programs specific to adolescents that are designed to stem the intergenerational transmission of domestic violence.

This chapter focuses primarily on a group intervention for male adolescents who have been abusive toward family members and/or in dating relationships. Some adolescents are court-ordered, while others are referred through youth diversion programs, schools, health care providers, child welfare services, mental health providers, and family members. The curriculum includes educational material and group exercises that assist in preventing further abuse by promoting attitudes and behaviors that support self-awareness and self-esteem, personal responsibility, empathy, healthy communication, nonviolent conflict resolution, and positive relationships with peers in the group and with group therapists. An overview of the intake and assessment process and the 14-week curriculum are provided. The chapter concludes with a brief look at program evaluation and offers suggestions for future research.

The adolescent treatment program presented in this chapter, called the Emerging Young Men's Program, was developed from our work with male adolescents at the Domestic Abuse Project (DAP) in Minneapolis, Minnesota. The Domestic Abuse Project was founded in 1979 as a response to requests from abused women who needed services in addition to shelter. Since then, DAP's services have increased to include programs for children and adolescents exposed to domestic violence, for men who abuse, for women who are violent in intimate relationships, and for male adolescents who are abusive toward family members and/or in dating relationships. The Emerging Young Men's Program has been in existence since 1990.

DESCRIPTION OF THE PROGRAM

The Emerging Young Men's Program uses structured education as well as dialogue and experiential (here-and-now) interventions within the group to facilitate behavioral and psychological change (changes in perceptions, attitudes, beliefs, emotions, cognitions). Interventions are designed to provide information so that adolescents can make healthy behavioral choices and as a means of preventing further abuse.

Using group therapy rather than individual therapy has several advantages. In general, group therapy reduces the sense of isolation, offers a healthy balance between adult authority and adolescent independence (providing an emotionally and physically safe environment while encouraging adolescents to "try on" new behaviors), offers a greater comfort level than individual therapy (the balance of power is spread among members rather than centralized in one adult), provides a safe place to learn and practice relationship skills, and offers a peer group in which to build a positive ego or sense of self (Carrell, 2000).

THEORETICAL AND
PHILOSOPHICAL FOUNDATIONS

Interventions in this model are grounded in cognitive-behavioral, social learning, feminist, developmental, and trauma theory. The philosophy of the adolescent treatment program at DAP is based on the following core beliefs:

- *Domestic violence is learned* from the family, community, neighborhood, and various social and cultural messages and attitudes that reinforce violence as acceptable behavior.
- *Violence is a chosen behavior* on the part of the violent person.
- *Violence is often motivated out of the desire for power and control*—even though other causes may be given.
- *Violence or other forms of abuse are not acceptable ways to control another person, to release stress, or to express feelings*—even in situations of self-defense, we teach that it is better to learn alternative ways to keep oneself safe.
- *Violence prevention* requires focusing on and promoting attitudes and behaviors that support the development of healthy, nonviolent relationships.

GROUP GOALS

We have identified six primary, interdependent treatment goals, along with several process and outcome goals for our treatment model. Process goals are specific activities designed to maximize goal attainment, and result in outcomes related to positive changes in both internal and external behavior. The outcome goals reflect achievement of the six primary group goals.

Goal 1: Having a Positive Group Experience

A positive group experience is critical to the success of the group and a precondition to the achievement of the other major goals. The process goals and outcome goals are:

- Positive interactions with peers and facilitators ("I feel respected and cared about.")
- Informed consent ("I willingly participate.")
- Maintaining group rules ("I feel safe and supported.")
- Playfulness, humor; having a snack ("Group is a fun experience.")

Goal 2: Stopping Abusive Behavior

The ultimate goal is that participants be nonviolent after completing our program. Some participants do make major changes in their behavior, choosing nonviolence as a way of interacting with their world, while others make less significant shifts in their overt behavior. The process goals and outcome goals are:

- Defining abuse ("Abuse is not okay.")
- Identifying feelings ("It is okay to feel and express my feelings appropriately.")
- Learning assertive communication ("I can be strong without being abusive.")
- Learning conflict resolution skills ("I can get my needs met without being abusive.")
- Developing STOP and Time-Out Plan ("I have the choice and ability to act in nonviolent ways.")

Goal 3: Taking Personal Responsibility for One's Thoughts, Feelings, and Actions

We seek to assist adolescents in taking responsibility for their thoughts, feelings, beliefs, attitudes, and overt behavior, teaching that we believe this responsibility leads to a more fulfilling and productive life. The process goals and outcome goals are:

- Identifying and expressing thoughts and feelings ("I have a responsibility to myself and to others to communicate assertively.")
- Developing STOP and Time-Out Plan ("I am responsible for my behavior.")
- Identifying and working on weekly goals ("I am successful in making changes in my life.")
- Completing and sharing written assignments with the group ("I am courageous enough to take responsibility for my thoughts, feelings, attitudes, perceptions, and behaviors.")

Goal 4: Strengthening Self-Esteem

As examined in Chapter 2, children who witness domestic violence are at risk for emotional, behavioral, social, school, and other problems, including problems in the area of self-esteem (see reviews in Edleson, 1999, and Holden, 1998). The process goals and outcome goals are:

- Positive interactions with peers and facilitators ("I am a good person and people like and respect me.")
- Setting and obtaining weekly goals ("I am capable of making changes in my life.")
- Learning and implementing new skills ("I am capable of interact-

ing respectfully toward others. I deserve to be treated respectfully and I treat others respectfully.")

Goal 5: Developing Insight

Self-awareness is a precursor to making personal changes. The process goals and outcome goals are:

- Identifying feelings ("I am aware of my feelings.")
- Developing STOP Plan ("I am aware of my personal cues to an escalation.")
- Sharing personal experiences and receive feedback ("I am aware of how others perceive me.")
- Participating in group exercises and dialogue ("I am learning more about my thoughts, feelings, attitudes, beliefs, perceptions, desires, values, and behaviors.")

Goal 6: Developing Empathy

Difficulty with empathy is one of the effects of exposure to adult domestic violence (see review in Holden, 1998). The process goals and outcome goals are:

- Modeling of empathy by group therapists ("Other people understand me and accept me.")
- Participation in group exercises and dialogue ("I understand how others feel.")
- Integration of new information via educational material ("I understand how my behavior might affect others and how the behavior of others affects me.")

INTAKE

Telephone Interview

This is usually the first contact the adolescent's parent/guardian (referred to hereafter as the "parent") has with the program's staff. The overall goals of the phone interview are to (1) begin building a working alliance with the parent; (2) provide program information and information specific to the intake; and (3) determine if an intake is appropriate. It is sometimes difficult to determine the appropriateness of establishing the intake based on a relatively short conversation. We use the following guidelines in our decision process.

Intake Indicators

The adolescent is between the ages of 13 and 18; the adolescent has been or is currently abusive toward family members and/or in dating relationships; participation in the program will not jeopardize the safety of the adolescent or his mother (e.g., the mother's partner, who is abusive, opposes the adolescent's participation in a domestic violence program, therefore increasing the mother's and/or adolescent's risk for abuse).

Referral Indicators

The adolescent is reported to be suicidal or self-injurious; the adolescent is reported to exhibit extreme behaviors, such as total withdrawal and lack of communication, hearing voices, or seeing things that other people do not see or hear; there is knowledge or suspicion of sexual, physical, or ritualistic abuse, or other severe trauma that has not been assessed or treated (e.g., ongoing domestic violence in the parent/adult relationship); there is knowledge of chemical dependency with the recommendation for treatment, and the adolescent has not undergone chemical health treatment; the adolescent has language limitations or disabilities that cannot be accommodated by the agency (e.g., has a hearing impairment that necessitates an interpreter, does not speak the language spoken by staff, or has a physical impairment that prevents access to the premises); the adolescent's abusive behavior, as reported by the referring parent, is directed only at people outside the family (e.g., peers, strangers). If a decision is made to conduct the intake, careful judgment is required when making a decision about involving the adolescent's other parent in the intake when there has been violence in the relationship between the adolescent's parents. We exercise the option of interviewing the other parent at a different time. In this way, the other parent can contribute information and feel heard, which may reduce the probability of that parent sabotaging or undermining the adolescent's treatment. Likewise, we use the same discretion when we have information about abuse being directed at the adolescent by the abusive parent.

In-Person Intake Interview

A semistructured interview format allows us to obtain specific information that is helpful in determining if the adolescent can benefit from the psychoeducational group we provide, and what other, if any, resources are needed for the adolescent and his family. Areas we inquire about and assess include family history and relationships; academic status and peer relationships; adolescent's health/mental health/chemical use; parent's health/mental health/chemical use; adolescent's strengths/areas of resilience; adolescent's interests; adolescent's current work history; family strengths; adolescent's suicidal ideation/behavior or other self-destructive behavior; adolescent's history of abusive behavior; history of abuse witnessed by the adolescent; history of abuse directed at the adolescent; adolescent's future orientation; parent's goals for the adolescent; and adolescent's goals for himself.

Interview Structure

The intake is structured in two parts. At the beginning the therapist, the adolescent, and the adolescent's parent(s) are all present. At this time we provide an orientation to the organization, to the group, and the intake. Following the orientation, we interview the parent in the presence of the adolescent, then we conduct a separate interview with the adolescent. Use of this particular structure:

1. Provides an opportunity to "break the secret" of domestic violence.
2. Provides an opportunity to observe whether the adolescent is able to respect the boundaries established at the beginning of the intake.
3. Offers the adolescent privacy, which can serve as a bridge to developing a working relationship.
4. Provides a snapshot of the relationship between the parent and her son.
5. Provides an opportunity to educate and reframe perceptions that lead to unhealthy dynamics in the parent–adolescent relationship.

ASSESSMENT

Upon gathering information in the areas noted above and, in some cases, collateral information, we make a decision or recommendation regarding the adolescent's involvement in the psychoeducational group and/or other recommendations given. The following behavioral indicators guide our decision-making process:

Indicators for Admitting to Group

Group generally works best for those adolescents who: demonstrate at least minimal acknowledgment of their abusive behavior; have some ability for insight and abstract thinking; feel some remorse for their behavior; demonstrate some capacity for empathy; and show some motivation for change.

Indicators Against Admitting to Group

Group is contraindicated for adolescents who: are chemically dependent and have had no intervention in this area; are actively suicidal or homicidal; are actively psychotic; are autistic or have other pervasive developmental disorders; are severely depressed and noncommunicative; are sexual perpetrators victimizing younger children, including family members; are unable to read and write; are victims of ongoing physical or sexual abuse; are involved in extremely violent or antisocial behavior outside the family; lack sufficient impulse control to function in a group setting; have absolutely no regard for others; have inadequate defenses, making it impossible for them to tolerate a group; are too defensive, indicating they are not ready for group; and/or are experiencing severe posttraumatic stress symptoms.

We make every attempt to gather enough information from the outset to make assessments that are in the best interest of adolescents and their families. Our assessment process does not end at the intake; we continue to assess how the intervention is impacting group members throughout their group participation.

GROUP COMPOSITION

Making decisions about group participation at any given time includes looking at variables of group composition, some of which include size of group, age and developmental status, race and ethnicity, disabilities, and physical and sexual abuse histories.

GROUP STRUCTURE

Each group session generally follows the format below.

Check-In

Asking members to briefly check in provides group members an opportunity to share personal life experiences, thoughts, feelings, and perceptions in an atmosphere of acceptance. It also provides therapists with information about what is going on in the daily/weekly lives of group members, which consequently gives a context for how adolescents present in the group. This information may, in turn, alter some of the agenda for the day (e.g., for a client in a personal crisis) or may alter the course of an individual's treatment plan (e.g., recommending a psychiatric consultation based on ongoing reports of depressive symptoms).

Review of Last Week's Session

Asking members to provide a review of the previous week's material and processes encourages verbal participation, helps members get focused, and assists in the integration of group material.

Process Issues Related to Check-In, Including Work on Personal Goals

After everyone has checked in, members are asked to talk about conflicts/abuse that they witnessed or were a part of in or outside of their families. Therapists use this as an opportunity to model supportive, empathetic feedback, and intervene in various ways to foster group interactions and creative problem solving.

Educational Component/Activity/Discussion

There is a topic and related activity for each session, as well as discussion related to what members learned and how this information applies to their lives.

Break

This gives members an opportunity to move and stretch their bodies, use the restroom, step outside to get fresh air, and talk with and develop closer relationships with one another.

Personal Goal Development

Each week, members identify, in writing, at least one behavioral goal (e.g., complete math homework; take out garbage without being asked) and one "self-care" goal (e.g., playing basketball, going for a walk, seeing a movie, listening to favorite music). Therapists assist members in establishing realistic goals in the service of "setting group members up for success." Personal and other barriers related to goal attainment are discussed, as well as efforts and achievements acknowledged.

Summary of Group

Group members summarize the events and group processes. Therapists use this opportunity to make observations about what they saw and heard in the group, give positive feedback, as well as state changes they would like the group to work on.

Check-Out

The purpose of check-out is for members to state how they were impacted by the group. Members are also asked to think in a discerning way about their participation in the group, and to make conscious decisions about how they want to participate the following week.

OVERVIEW OF GROUP SESSIONS

The following is a brief description of the 14-week program; each session is 2 hours in length. The sessions are ordered in the manner we found most logical, however, we have changed the order of material on many occasions, based on the needs of each group.

Session 1: Introduction and Definitions of Abuse

The desired outcomes of the first session include establishing the group as a place where members feel physically and emotionally safe, and increasing the desire of members to attend and participate in the group. During this session, the facilitators give participants information about the program, provide role clarification and expectations of therapists and group members, and have the group revisit the concepts of confidentiality and limits to confidentiality to assure a clear understanding. (These concepts should be discussed at intake.) Group members and therapists also participate in developing group rules as well as sharing information about themselves.

Session 2: How I Learned to Be Abusive

The desired outcomes for participants include understanding that domestic violence is learned and socially sanctioned, that there are alternatives to being abusive, and that violence happens in other households. We have found that using a film or video is one of the best ways to initiate this learning and to challenge the belief or perception of being the only one who has grown up with violence. Therapists help members identify and acknowledge the consequences for the victims of domestic violence, as well as their minimization and/or denial of the impact that witnessing violence has on individuals, including themselves.

Session 3: Payoffs and Consequences—A Look at Power and Control

Desired outcomes for participants include increased awareness of payoffs and consequences for abusive behavior, increased awareness of potential effects of witnessing domestic abuse, increased capacity for empathy, and ability to differentiate between appropriate and inappropriate expressions of anger. We provide members with a definition of *payoffs* (something that usually happens right after the abuse that reinforces abusive behavior and is usually experienced as short-term; for example, getting revenge, getting what you want, getting the last word in, feeling powerful and in control) and *consequences* (negative results related to abusive behavior, such as losing a friend/girlfriend, being grounded, being on probation, getting physically injured, getting kicked out of school). A recurrent theme is helping adolescents understand that they always have control over how they respond to any situation. Additionally, sharing how we have dealt with feelings of powerlessness is another way to role-model positive, creative problem resolution by focusing on what we can do differently as opposed to attempting to change others.

Session 4: STOP Plan

Desired outcomes for participants include developing an understanding of the escalation process of abuse, understanding that escalations can occur over varying time periods, increased awareness of the motivations underlying abusive behavior, becoming aware of personal situations, thoughts, verbal expressions, and physical and emotional cues that precede abusive behavior, and increasing awareness of the interconnections between emotions, thoughts, images, and bodily reactions. We ask members to participate in a guided imagery exercise to increase bodily awareness. We ask members to pay attention to their breathing and what is going on with their bodies (sensations, thoughts, feelings, movements). We talk with members about the value of self-awareness related to what is going on internally and externally, which helps in managing one's emotions and behaviors. Information is provided on the progression of violence and on identification of cues related to the STOP Plan (*Situations*—circumstances, or scenarios when one typically gets angry; *Thinking*—negative things one says about the situation, about the people involved in the situation or about oneself; *Out Loud*—what one says out loud before acting abusively: putdowns, swearing, threats, and name calling are considered abusive and not part of the buildup; and *Physical/Emotional*—voluntary and involuntary bodily sensations or behaviors indicating one is feeling angry). Once group members grasp the concept of cues involved in the escalation process, we ask them to complete the STOP worksheet, which requires them to identify personal cues related to these areas. Members then share their written cues with the group.

Session 5: Time-Out Plan

Desired outcomes for participants include gaining an understanding of the varying levels of cues (low, medium, high), rating personal cues according to the progression of abuse and determining when to take a time-out, developing and sharing with the group a personalized Time-Out Plan, and helping group members prepare for the upcoming family session. We describe *low-level cues* as typically related to everyday stressors, including frustration and irritability; if experienced in isolation, these stressors would be manageable, but when combined they play a part in the escalation. *Medium-level cues* are often associated with interpersonal conflict or incidents that challenge one's self-image or negatively affect their view of themselves. Individuals often feel on the edge of abuse with medium-level cues. *High-level cues* indicate a "high-risk" time when one easily moves into more aggressive thoughts, images, and verbalizations. Group members use the cues written on their STOP worksheet to complete their Cue Rating Worksheet. Members identify when they need to take a time-out based on their personal cues. We help participants see how taking a time-out when experiencing low- and medium-level cues is most effective, and leaves them feeling in charge of their emotions and behaviors. Members complete a Time-Out Plan, which includes identifying places where they can go to calm down, what they will do to help themselves deescalate, people they can talk to about what is upsetting them, specific positive self-talk they will engage in to help them manage their emotions, and what they will do on a regular basis to help themselves manage and prevent stress.

Preparation for the family session includes identifying participants, giving members a preview of the upcoming session, and discussion related to members' associated feelings, all of which serves to alleviate anticipated uncomfortable emotions. Providing a clear picture of what will take place helps reduce anxiety and gives adolescents an opportunity to plan and problem solve. Creative suggestions from peers and therapists can help members better manage their emotions and behavior prior to the family session.

Session 6: Family Session

Desired outcomes for the family session include establishing the agenda and boundaries of the Family Session, keeping a dialogue open between participants and the therapists, assessing how the intervention is working, discussing the STOP worksheet and Time-Out Plan, reviewing the educational material discussed in group, providing support for the adolescent, providing general feedback about the group member's participation and providing support for parents/caregivers or partners. Therapists often state the primary focus of each session and ask the adolescent to fill in with additional details and his personal learning experiences. We ask the adolescent to share his entire Time-Out Plan so that all parties are "in the know," which is necessary for others to be able to support his plan. We solicit feedback from his family members and/or partners regarding their ability to support the Time-Out Plan. We ask the adolescent to talk about how he thinks he is doing in group, what is helpful and not helpful, and what else, if anything, he wants or needs from the therapists in regard to his group participation or from family members or from his intimate partner. We solicit feedback from parents or partners regarding how the group member is making use of the group intervention and what changes in attitude and/or behavior they have witnessed. We give general feedback about the member's participation in the group.

Session 7: Emotions

Desired outcomes for adolescents include increased ability to experience and label emotions, learning that all feelings are okay, knowing it is okay to appropriately express all feelings in group, increased awareness of the impact of gender socialization, and learning that people experience more than one emotion at a time. The activity for Session 7 begins with an educational component related to gender socialization, followed by an expressive arts exercise. We use a relaxation exercise followed by guided imagery to help members see and experience two emotions, *anger* and a *painful or stress-producing emotion*. These internal images associated with the emotions are then expressed through drawing. After completing both drawings, group members share what they have drawn and share personal insights related to this experience. It is particularly helpful for the male group therapist to be adept at expressing his own emotions in order to model this for the group.

Session 8: Styles of Communication

Desired outcomes for adolescents include increasing self-awareness through guided imagery, understanding of four different styles of communication (assertive, passive, aggressive, and passive-aggressive), and applying these concepts by identifying their own personal styles of communication and how their style might change under various circumstances and with different people. We use selected scenarios or role plays as a way for adolescents to practice identifying the different styles of communication; the adolescents observe who is engaging in what style of communication and when. Group members also complete a written worksheet that asks them to apply these concepts to their personal life. We ask members to establish a goal for the upcoming week related to modifying their communication style with one person. We teach that being assertive helps people to feel more in charge of their lives and can boost their self-esteem since it requires taking responsibility for expressing personal thoughts, feelings, needs, and desires.

Session 9: Conflict Resolution

Desired outcomes for adolescents include increased insight/awareness of thoughts/images, feelings, and bodily sensations through the use of guided imagery, increased knowledge and practice of conflict resolution skills and assertive communication, and increased ability for empathy. We connect the value of increased self-awareness to the STOP and Time-Out Plans, which help participants manage emotions, thoughts, and behaviors. We also explore beliefs and attitudes about conflict— common beliefs we encounter are that *conflict is bad* and *conflict means violence/abuse is inevitable*. We use role plays that challenge members to try on assertive communication; this is followed by group discussion.

Session 10: Gender Role Socialization

Desired outcomes for adolescents include listening to their own inner wisdom/voice through the use of guided imagery in problem solving, gaining an understanding of the concept of gender role, understanding that stereotypical gender role socialization gives permission for gender-based violence, gaining an understanding of payoffs and consequences of maintaining stereotypical gender role behavior, and gaining insight into payoffs and consequences of nontraditional gender role attitudes and behaviors. Members identify problems they are having trouble working out and then participate in a guided imagery exercise in which they imagine meeting a helper who is their inner guide, which is, in fact, their own inner wisdom. We help members understand that we are asking them to listen to their own hearts, that their inner guide is their own truth speaking to them. We use a film or a group exercise that challenges members to understand and think critically about gender role socialization and to gain insight into how their own socialization has been impacted by the messages they received from significant sources (e.g., family, church, school/peers, television, media).

Session 11: Dating Violence

Desired outcomes for adolescents include understanding how gender role socialization plays out in dating relationships, challenging one's own thinking about cultural myths related to dating relationships, learning early warning signs of abusive relationships, and learning characteristics of healthy relationships. We use a video followed by questions and discussion related to gender role attitudes, beliefs, and behaviors of the abusive character(s) in the video. We help members focus on the underlying attitudes and beliefs of identified abusive behavior and nonabusive/healthy behavior. We remind participants that they, like other males, are at risk for abusing intimate partners by the sheer fact that they have been socialized in this culture, and even more so if they grew up witnessing domestic violence. We inform members that next week will in some way be their last typical group, since the following week is their family session.

Session 12: Taking Responsibility for My Abusive Behavior

Desired outcomes for adolescents include identifying the victim(s) of their abuse, taking ownership of their abusive behavior, identifying cues of the escalation that preceded the abuse, identifying the results of the abuse, feeling the emotions related to a specific incident and conveying these honestly to the group, relaying how they would behave differently in similar situations using their current STOP and Time-Out Plans, and listening to feedback from peers and therapists. The written exercise, Taking Responsibility for My Abusive Behavior, is designed to incorporate previous learning into a personalized account of a specific abusive incident. It allows members the opportunity to reconstruct the incident using their STOP and Time-Out Plans, which become the basis of learning how to make better choices in the future. Upon completion, members share their written work and receive feedback from peers and therapists. We remind members that next week is the family session and the week following is their final session.

Session 13: Family Session

The desired outcomes for the family session include assessing how the intervention is working, providing continued support for all family members/intimate partners, providing feedback regarding the adolescent's group participation, and providing recommendations regarding future services if needed. Lastly, we discuss the upcoming research, reminding parents and adolescents that we will be contacting them 6 and 12 months from now. We provide parents with a positive portrait of their son, as well as noting his struggles in the group and areas he needs to work on. We ask adolescents to provide feedback about their group experience. We solicit feedback from parent(s) regarding positive changes their son has made. We also inquire about current or ongoing conflicts, about his use of time-outs, about ongoing abusive behavior, or other concerns parents or partners might have. We also review the concept of a time-out and the adolescent's specific plan for taking a time-out.

Session 14: Closure/Celebration

The desired outcomes for adolescents include reviewing the educational content of the group, sharing personal thoughts and feelings related to the group, providing feedback to group therapists in the form of a written evaluation, and saying good-bye to peers and group therapists. We keep the atmosphere of the final group casual and fun. We celebrate with food that group members previously selected. When reviewing group material, therapists lead the discussion, asking members about key points and learning they gained from each session. Following this, we ask members to share personal and meaningful experiences related to group and complete a written evaluation. We select a closing ceremony that fits the overall group dynamic. For example, when we have a group that advances to a "working stage," we might close with having each group member identify one thing they liked about each person or how each person helped them, and put this in writing so they can all leave with something material as a reminder of the group. Therapists also participate in the closing ceremony by providing each group member with positive feedback or a gift that represents the theme of the group or something more personal to each member (e.g., inspirational words, printed or engraved on stones).

PROGRAM EVALUATION

Throughout the group process, we encourage members to give us feedback about the group and how they are impacted by their group participation. Likewise, we ask and encourage feedback from parents. Additionally, we obtain written feedback from members who have completed group. Members rate themselves (Likert scale) on their accomplishment of the six primary group goals and the associated process goals noted earlier. Members also provide additional qualitative feedback about their overall group experience. Although this feedback is limited in scope, it does suggest that most members have benefited from their group experience, accomplishing the identified goals and emphasizing the importance of the group processes and their personal relationships with the therapists and group members.

We recognize the limitations of the feedback from members, and consequently are in the process of developing follow-up research with adolescents and their parents and/or intimate partners. This follow-up research will evaluate cognitive, emotional, social, and behavioral changes, 6 and 12 months following completion of group. This research will be both qualitative and quantitative in nature. Group therapists are also using an engagement measure to examine how engagement in the group processes impacts current and future change in the areas noted above.

SUMMARY AND CONCLUSIONS

Due to limited programming and research in the area of youth and domestic violence, many questions remain unanswered. Some recommendations for further exploration include the following:

• Expanded research is needed to examine various models for group intervention with youth who engage in domestic violence to develop effective intervention and prevention programs. This research needs to consider variables including, but not limited to, age and developmental status, gender, mental status/diagnosis, cultural differences, type and extent of abusive behavior engaged in by adolescents, and type and level of involvement of parents in their adolescent's treatment.

• Research is needed to examine and define vital group processes that assist in achieving identified group and personal goals. A closer look at the cotherapy relationship, for example, may offer valuable information. Use of qualitative research can provide an in-depth evaluation of the processes and quality of the program that can be used to improve program effectiveness.

• We need to gain a better understanding of how personal and situational mediating factors influence the adolescent's ability to function in and outside of the group. For example, personal mediating variables include, but are not limited to, having an internal or external locus of control, temperament, level of social competence, deficiencies in basic academic skills, academic success or special talents, adolescent's mental health status, substance abuse, capacity for empathy, and beliefs about who is responsible for the violence in the family. Likewise, situational mediating factors include, but are not limited to, disrupted routines and homelessness, poverty, availability and accessibility of local social support and helping agencies, continued interparental physical and/or verbal aggression, divorce and visitation conflicts, status of parent–adolescent relationships, mental health status of parents, parent's substance abuse, parent-to-adolescent verbal and/or physical aggression, exposure to school and community violence, and positive relationship(s) with others in and/or outside the family. The presence or absence of both personal and situational variables tends to be either risk-enhancing or protective in nature and has the potential to influence the adolescent's ability to use the educational material and take part in group exercises and dialogue. When combined, these variables result in complex dynamics that need to be considered when evaluating treatment models to determine what model is most beneficial for which individuals.

• Further exploration and evaluation of collaborations is called for in the area of youth domestic violence. This requires identifying key stakeholders or multiple service systems and organizations that share common goals (e.g., juvenile court judges, police, probation officers, child welfare agencies, educational systems, youth diversion programs, family court, health and mental health systems, particularly those servicing children and adolescents, domestic violence service organizations, restorative justice programs, culturally specific community organizations and community leaders, religious communities, family and extended family members).

• Research needs to address the unintended results of intervention and prevention programs and how these unintended results may impact the adolescent, the group dynamics, and family dynamics. Although the intention is for adolescents to experience group as a safe place to disclose internal and external life experiences, we find that participation in the group is also a stressful event not only for the adolescent but the family as well. Researchers and helping professionals working with this population need to be conscious of these and other unintended results in program development and implementation.

REFERENCES

Carrell, S. (2000). *Group exercises for adolescents: A manual for therapists.* Thousand Oaks, CA: Sage.

Edleson, J. L. (1999). Children's witnessing of adult domestic violence. *Journal of Interpersonal Violence, 14,* 839–870.

Holden, G. W. (1998). Introduction: The development of research into another consequence of family violence. In G. W. Holden, R. Geffner, & E. N. Jouriles (Eds.), *Children exposed to marital violence: Theory, research, and applied issues* (pp. 1–18). Washington DC: American Psychological Association.

Wolfe, D. A., & Jaffe, P. G. (2001). Prevention of domestic violence: Emerging initiatives. In S. A. Graham-Bermann & J. L. Edleson (Eds.), *Domestic violence in the lives of children: The future of research, intervention, and social policy* (pp. 283–298). Washington DC: American Psychological Association.

Part II

INDIVIDUAL- AND
GROUP-LEVEL RESPONSES

5

Fostering Resilient Coping in Children Exposed to Violence

Cultural Considerations

SANDRA A. GRAHAM-BERMANN and HILDA M. HALABU

Immigration is a common experience for American children. Twenty percent of all children in the United States are children of immigrants, and 48% of children in New York City schools come from immigrant-headed households (Suarez-Orozco, 2000). (See Chapter 9 for a discussion of immigration from a Canadian perspective.) The economic and social burdens of racism affect all children of color and their families, either directly or indirectly. Yet, ethnic minority children and immigrant children vary in terms of risk factors and degree of acculturation. The stress of immigration is associated with a loss of social group, status, the process of acculturation, and the trauma of violence either witnessed or experienced by children during or after their migration (Espin, 1987; Garcia-Coll & Magnuson, 1997; Sluzki, 1979). These facts suggest that the mental health needs of minority children are significant and varied.

The needs of minority children exposed to violence have yet to be determined.

Poor families and ethnic minority families are disproportionately represented among those who receive services in shelters and in community-based programs for abused women and their children (Root, 1996; Sampson, 1993). To date, the literature on designing and evaluating intervention programs for children exposed to domestic violence largely leaves culture and ethnicity out of the picture. Yet, we know from researchers who study ethnicity and interventions for adults in other contexts that culturally appropriate programs enhance the efficacy of the intervention and improve outcomes (U.S. Surgeon General, 2001; Zane, Hall, Sue, Young, & Nunez, 2002). For example, Castillo (1997) noted four ways in which culture can impact interventions for adults:

1. Taking culture into account in fashioning interventions
2. Understanding the subjective experience of a family's ethnicity and culture
3. Identifying cultural constructions of the problem
4. Using culturally appropriate methods and measures to evaluate outcomes

However, in our experience, adult models differ substantially from the ways in which culture and ethnicity appear and play out in interventions designed for children. The role of culture and ethnicity in children's interventions is just beginning to be explored.

In this chapter, we will consider a number of issues related to culture and ethnicity and their implications for designing and implementing intervention programs for children exposed to domestic violence. More particularly, we will illustrate the ways in which culture and ethnicity are part of two intervention programs that enhance children's recovery from trauma and foster resilience in the face of violence: The Kids' Club and Preschool Kids' Club programs (Graham-Bermann, 1992; Graham-Bermann & Follett, 1999; Graham-Bermann & Halabu, 2001). Both are 10-week interventions that target 3- to 13-year-old children's knowledge about domestic violence, their attitudes and beliefs about families and domestic violence, their fears and worries, and their social behavior in the small-group setting.

CULTURE AND EXPOSURE TO DOMESTIC VIOLENCE

Defining Domestic Violence

Domestic violence is defined here as incidents of both mild and severe violence by one intimate adult partner with another. Children are considered to be exposed to domestic violence when they are present as eye-witnesses, when they overhear the abuse taking place, or when they are present during the aftermath of violence (e.g., arrest of perpetrator, emergency room visits, descriptions of what took place when police arrive, moving to a shelter, etc.).

Defining Cultural Competence

According to Sue (1998), cultural competence (along with the broader concept of multiculturalism) is the belief that people should not only appreciate and recognize other cultural groups but also be able to effectively work with them. To competently serve a diverse set of clients and to achieve credibility, in this case with children from different minority groups, it is essential to learn about each individual's culture and to be sensitive and flexible in interacting with the children (Porterotto, Casas, Suzuki, & Alexander, 1995; Sue, 1998).

Culture and Children's Violence Exposure

It is well known that poverty and exposure to violence are often entwined (Sampson, 1993). While women and children across all ethnic groups and social classes can be subjugated by more powerful males, we are just beginning to appreciate the increased risk of domestic violence victimization for women of color (O'Keefe, 1994a). In some studies, poor children and children of color are exposed to disproportionately higher levels of violence in both their communities and at home than nonminority children (Bell & Chance-Hill, 1991). Clearly, as the research shows, domestic violence is but one of many factors, including poverty and immigrant status, to affect ethnically diverse families (Kanuha, 1994).

Very few studies have specifically examined the relationships between ethnicity and the cultural context of the families of children exposed to domestic violence. Three studies that take ethnicity into account show that Caucasian children score higher on conduct and aggression problems than do African American children exposed to the abuse of their mothers (O'Keefe, 1994b; Stagg, Wills, & Howell, 1989; Westra & Martin, 1981). Another study found similar results—namely, the adjustment of children of abused women differed by race. African American children and their mothers were less likely to describe themselves as having serious problems in adjustment than Caucasian children exposed to similar amounts of domestic violence (Graham-Bermann & Gruber, 2003). These studies suggest that children have different needs when entering treatment. Still, this body of research provides scant evidence of the specific needs of children of color following violence exposure. It is important to note here that children of color who do not present with obvious psychopathology or serious problems in adjustment may develop problems later, and, conversely, children's adjustment problems may abate over time. Thus, all children can benefit from education and intervention programs.

CULTURALLY APPROPRIATE INTERVENTIONS FOR CHILDREN

Interventions for children exposed to violence can and do serve children from diverse cultural and ethnic groups. Cultural considerations arise at every stage in the process, from who attends the intervention program, who the group leaders will be, how they will be trained, and which topics are addressed and in what ways.

Description of the Programs

Two intervention programs that enhance children's recovery from trauma and foster resilience in the face of violence are The Kids' Club and Preschool Kids' Club programs. The programs are based on social learning theory and social cognition theory, where some children are considered to have developed distorted paradigms of gender roles, interpersonal relationships, and social skills following exposure to violence (Graham-Bermann, 1998; Graham-Bermann & Brescoll, 2000). In addition, many children exposed to violence are known to suffer symptoms of traumatic stress (Graham-Bermann & Levendosky, 1998; Rossman & Ho, 2000). Thus, program goals include reducing children's anxiety, building appropriate coping skills and defenses, as well as enhancing social skill and pride in the family. Children who participate in these programs typically present with distress and anxiety, as well as aggression. The 10 sessions cover the following topics: becoming a group; identifying feelings and managing feelings associated with violence; responsibility for violence; identifying fears and worries connected with violence; safety planning; gender roles in families; family strengths and weaknesses; conflict resolution strategies; lessons learned; and processing termination of the group. A Mothers' Empowerment Program that focuses on parenting support for abused women is offered in conjunction with the children's programs in both shelter and community settings (Graham-Bermann & Levendosky, 1994).

Groups generally consist of from three to seven children, and include children similar in age from both genders. There are two leaders for each group who receive weekly supervision of their work. During supervision, the group leaders are trained in ethical issues, cultural issues, and doing psychotherapy with children exposed to violence. Many steps are taken to enhance treatment fidelity for these programs, including extensive training and supervision of therapists/service providers and the construction of standard treatment manuals. (A more comprehensive description of these programs is available on the web page *www.sandragb.com*).

Recognizing the Multicultural Context

Over the past 12 years, The Kids' Club program has often consisted of participants from more than one or two ethnic groups, and families with disparate constraints and resources in their lives. For example, in one group, there were five children, from African American, Irish American, Italian American, Jamaican, and Asian immigrant families. Their mothers ranged in age from 26 to 39, and the children had between one and four siblings. While they all shared the common experience of exposure to their mother's abuse, four out of five children did not live with their biological fathers, and three had a new father figure in the home. Some of their mothers had jobs, while others were looking for work. Some still had contact with the abuser on a regular basis, and others had moved away. One mother was currently being stalked and threatened. All lived in community settings rather than in a shelter, although two families had been to a shelter before.

Since the children of abused women who participate in intervention programs vary in their family circumstances, an appreciation of the diverse contexts of the children's lives is essential. In this case, group leaders can enhance their ability to relate to each child and to establish credibility by learning more about the family's circumstances and cultural context. The subjective experience of culture includes both what the individual child identifies as important in her or his own culture as well as how the child perceives the cultural identity of others.

The Role of the Therapist

Empowering interventions should be fashioned in such a way that the participant is able to tell his or her own story, to identify and build upon existing strengths, and to enhance his or her power and coping (Gutierrez, 1990). The therapist's task is to bring to light the unique and shared experiences of groups of children exposed to violence. Culture is used in the service of making sense of at least some parts of the experience and how to cope with it—in this case, exposure to violence. When working with minority clients, it is especially important that the therapist take an active stance that encourages and includes the children rather than a passive or neutral stance that can create wariness and anxiety (Allen, 1996). To facilitate comfort and cultural awareness, the group leader must be able to assume an empathic stance and be open to exploring cultural issues when they arise, but also to know how to avoid cultural stereotyping and overgeneralization. This adaptability has been referred to as "dynamic sizing" by Sue (1998), who describes the ways in which effective therapists know "when to generalize and be inclusive and when to individualize and be exclusive" while still appreciating the salience of culture in intervention. These issues are pertinent whether groups are heterogeneous or consist of children from only one cultural group.

Opportunities naturally arise in the course of the children's programs where culture may be introduced and discussed. The following example illustrates how issues of diversity were brought into the very first session of The Kids' Club curriculum. After one group of 6- to 9-year-olds gathered in their meeting room, they made name tags to help introduce themselves to one another and drew pictures of things they liked and disliked. One group member could not quite guess the identity of a graduate student group leader who was from Pakistan. This African American boy asked her, "But what *are* you?" (Children are often blunt in asking questions about ethnicity or when satisfying their curiosity about differences.) It took the group leader a few moments to figure out what he wanted to know. When she mentioned her country of origin, he said he had never heard of it. She told the group about where her family had come from. This started a conversation about the cultural background of other children in the group. One girl volunteered that her mother was from Mexico but she was born in New York. Another child spoke of her Italian grandfather. Several children were African American, yet originated from different places—for example, one was born in Jamaica, two came from families that originated in Africa. A few children were unsure of their family background, but offered that they came from other states. The original question gave the group leaders a chance, in the second session, to bring in a world map to show the children where their families might have lived. The group leaders' flexibility and responsiveness to a child's curiosity provided an opportunity for the children in this group to learn about and to enjoy their cultural backgrounds.

In a different group, one leader was of Korean American descent. The children were genuinely interested in where her family came from and whether she was "white" or not. One girl even challenged her when she said that she was an American. In both groups, the leaders took the opportunity to talk about cultural background and diversity to expand the children's understanding of these categories. Lively discussions ensued about each child's family of origin in both groups. In general, young children are more likely to ask direct questions, whereas older children may have more information to share concerning their family's origins. The combination of enthusiasm and natural curiosity prompted these discussions of cultural diversity. As each child described his or her own culture and context, it was evident that there were individual differences among families in acculturation (Dana, 1993). Similarly, children within the same cultural group varied considerably in their experiences. The goal of the first sessions in both children's programs is to help them to "become a group." The adaptability of the group leaders and discussion of diversity fostered this goal.

Matching Client and Therapist Ethnicity

One prominent issue in research on adults in therapy is whether it is best to have service providers from the same cultural or ethnic group as the service recipient. The policy of pairing group leaders' ethnicity with the ethnicity of children within a particular group naturally brings questions of culture into the design of the program. There is a range of opinion as to whether the therapist or evaluator should be someone from the same culture (Sue, 1988; Jones, 1989) and under what conditions this pairing is most important to the client. For example, studies of Asian American adult clients demonstrate that the degree of fit in terms of cognitive match between the client and the therapist determines therapeutic success. Clients are more satisfied and have better therapeutic outcomes when they share a similar construction of the problem (Sue, 1988). Conversely, Helms (1990) found that not all African American clients preferred African American therapists but that those who did had a stronger identity as African American.

However, as Sue (1988) points out, the

> ethnicity of the therapist or client and ethnic match are distal variables; consequently, weak or conflicting results are likely to be found between ethnic match and outcome. Ethnicity per se tells us very little about the attitudes, values, experiences and behavior of individuals, therapists or clients who interact in a therapy session. What is known is that although groups exhibit cultural differences, considerable individual differences may exist within groups. Ethnic matches can result in cultural mismatches if therapists and clients from the same ethnic group show markedly different values. (p. 305)

Conversely, ethnic mismatches do not necessarily imply cultural mismatches, because therapists and clients from different ethnic groups may share similar values, lifestyles, and experiences.

When we first began the intervention programs described here, we thought it best to match the ethnicity of the child who receives services with the ethnicity of at least one of the two group leaders or service providers, to facilitate the child's comfort and enhance a sense of empowerment. Over the years, we have been fortunate to have a varied group of graduate students who serve as group leaders when implementing The Kids' Club programs. Approximately half of these students are women of color and international students. We thought that the group leaders would serve as role models in the comfortable exchange of information and leading activities that explore family context and culture. However, the reality is that The Kids' Club programs now take place in a number of different settings, states, and countries. The group leaders vary from graduate students at universities, program providers in shelters, to social workers and psychologists in medical and mental health clinics. Similarly, the populations of children who participate in these programs vary from those in one cultural group to those in multicultural and multilingual communities.

In many cases, intervention is usually offered to abused women and their children in communities or shelters on a first-come, first-served basis, without regard to the match of ethnicity either within the group or between client and helper. Thus, a more salient issue, if language is not a barrier, is having someone experienced in cultural diversity, a knowledgeable therapist who is an empathic and engaging listener, and someone who can be respected by a diverse group of clients, be they adults or children (Gutierrez, 1990; Bell & Mattis, 2000; Parham, 2002).

Culturally Appropriate Interventions

A second matching issue is agreement about the appropriateness of the intervention. A number of researchers show that when the adult client and therapist agree on what are acceptable solutions to the problem, there is greater treatment success (Kleinman, 1992; Zane et al., 2002). In general, researchers find that it is most important for the ethnicity of the client to match the ethnicity of the helper when the language is different from that of the majority (Sue, 1988). One example is The Moms Helping Kids Program (Hokoda, Edleson, Tate, Carter, & Guerrero, 1998) designed for the special needs of Latino abused mothers who are primarily Spanish-speaking. Generally speaking, the cultural knowledge of the therapist is necessary to develop a good therapeutic alliance that enhances trust and thereby affects treatment outcomes. But the more important aspect is the ability to translate specific knowledge into practice. Sue (1988) states that "in the treatment of ethnic minority clients, a therapist's knowledge of the client's culture is distal to outcome in the sense that the cultural knowledge must somehow be translated into concrete behaviors in the therapy session. These culturally based behaviors may enhance the process of credibility (e.g., the client's belief that the therapist is understanding, knowledgeable and competent), which is more proximal to therapy outcome and effectiveness" (p. 305).

More specific to our purposes, sharing similar viewpoints, similar dilemmas, and similar solutions to problems with others from the same culture can provide a focal point to treatment that enhances social support and preserves an individual child's adjustment (Aponte, Rivers, & Wohl, 1994). Conversely, the absence of these recognized experiences and formats during stressful times is associated with isolation and emotional dysfunction, particularly for adults closer to the immigration generation (Tseng & Hsu, 1980). Ethnicity is described as an individual's embodiment and internalization of cultural tradition and preservation of cultural ways (Ogbu, 1990). It is important for children to feel connected with their cultural origins and ethnicity as well as to learn about the cultures of others.

Reinforcing Positive Associations to Culture

At several points in The Kids' Club programs, children engage in activities about their attitudes toward families and gender. These sessions often present opportunities to share a sense of identification with and pride in cultural background. The children's group leaders model cultural pride and, when appropriate, initiate discussions about cultural background and integrate cultural issues into the goals of each session. In the eighth session of the Preschool Kids' Club program for 3- to 5-year-olds, children show or tell what they like and dislike about families. The aim of this session is to encourage children to identify family strengths and to share their disappointments together. These goals can be achieved through a number of different activities planned by the group leaders. Activities that involve play are used as a natural way to promote healing for children following abuse or exposure to violence (Gil, 1991).

To draw out the issues of culture and cultural identity during a session about families, the leaders of one group cut out pictures from culturally appropriate magazines reflecting people from multiple ethnic groups—the same groups as the children's families—engaged in a range of activities. There were mothers, fathers, babies, children, and grandparents. Children selected among the cutout figures to make a collage of the people in their family. The children then presented their creations to others in the group and pointed out what they liked about being in their particular family. Group leaders can also comment directly on the cultural aspects and strengths of each child's family if that seems appropriate. Thus, it is possible for even young children to recognize that those in different families face similar problems and that families can also be a source of pride and strength (Graham-Bermann, 2001).

Recognizing Cultural Differences in Expression and Behavior

When planning activities that require children to participate and share in the expression of feelings, there are times when knowledge of cultural norms and expectations can be taken into account (Roopnarine, Johnson, & Hooper, 1994). For example, in some cultures there is a strong prohibition against the outward and public expression of feelings. In Native American and Asian American families, the overt expression of emotion is generally proscribed (Nguyen, 1992; Willis, Dobrec, & Sipes, 1992). Others have described some Asian American families as more likely to reflect than to take action, and more likely to keep anger and opinions inside when distressed (Ho, 1992). Concomitantly, African American children and Latino males have been described as acting out rather than holding in their frustrations (e.g., Allen & Majidi-Ahi, 1989; Ramirez, 1989; Weisz et al., 1993). It is essential that the therapist have a good grounding in cultural differences so as not to misunderstand the level of the child's participation and expression during group activities when such differences arise.

The goals of several Kids' Club program sessions are to have children identify alternative ways of resolving conflict, to identify and discuss the role of men and women in the family, and to enhance their capacity for coping with the violence in their lives. In one group of 11- to 13-year-old girls, the group leaders used a "Dear Renatta" task to elicit group members' responses to questions written by "preteens who had witnessed fighting in the family." This task allowed the children to respond through displacement and try out new ways of solving problems similar to the ones they faced at home. Along the way, children learned from each other in the context of being the "expert" who offered advice. One letter stated:

Dear Renatta:

I am stuck because in my house my dad won't let us tell anyone what goes on in our family. Sometimes it gets pretty rough and I get scared. What should I do?

Signed, Ateshia

In this mixed racial group, a Caucasian girl advised, "Just call the police." One African American girl shook her head and said, "No way. My mom doesn't want police in our house—*ever!*" Another biracial girl added, "The police won't even come into our neighborhood. So that's not gonna work. No one will help us out." "We are not supposed to tell anyone what happened," offered an Asian American child who said that her mom was afraid to get help because her grandmother is not yet living in this country. Next, a Latina girl said that she turns to her mother or grandmother when things get tough—"Mi abuela me escucha" ("My grandmother listens to me"). One African American girl said that her grandmother usually takes her to church. Clearly, children approach the task of coping with exposure to domestic violence through their own cultural lens and family experience. In this group, both strengths as well as limitations were discussed when coping with violence.

Recognizing Cultural Variation within and between Groups

Cultural factors also are clearly important to consider when designing intervention programs for children (Cohler, Stott, & Musick, 1995; Masten & Coatsworth, 1995). Variations within cultural groups should always be taken into account (Pope-Davis & Coleman, 2001). For example, there is no single cultural description of the "Black family" (Allen & Majidi-Ahi, 1989) in America, as African American families have emanated from a number of countries and continents. Still, studies show some common attributes of African American families. African American families tend to exert control over their children, emphasize moral and religious values, and have less openly expressed conflict than Caucasian and other ethnic family groups (Gillum, Gomez-Marin, & Prineas, 1984). African American mothers also teach their children to combat racism and work to enhance their child's self-esteem (Peters, 1981). Williams, Boggess, and Carter (2001) write of the challenges that many African American women and children face following family violence, with the competing interests of valuing the father in the family and trying to keep safe. Any consideration of the African American family has to take the ecological context into account in either weighing options or evaluating outcomes, as there is great variation in the social context of families. Thus, the dual roles of racism and lack of opportunity constrain the options that are available to many African American families.

Ideally, each child can be appreciated in terms of his or her own progress from the start to the end of the program, rather than compared with children in other cultural groups. This approach works well when assessing whether a child is coping adequately, particularly when the program has reasonable goals that reflect the cultural and situational experience of the child. However, there are times when knowledge of differences between cultural groups can profitably be taken into account in assessing the efficacy of an intervention program. As an example, when assessing adjustment in broad domains such as social functioning, academic achievement, socially appropriate conduct, and emotion regulation, it would be useful to know that children from Asian backgrounds tend to be more socially reticent and more emotionally restrained than children from Hispanic families (Paniagua, 1998). Similarly, it is crucial that the evaluator be aware of the level of acculturation of the child and family, including the primary language spoken at home. Where appropriate, assessments should be done in the child's native language.

Adapting the Program to Local Needs

To provide maximum flexibility, the content of program sessions may be adapted to fit the cultural setting. For example, in another session, a list of options was created by a group for what some children can do when there is fighting in the family. Responses for a group of 5- to 7-year-olds included "telling someone else," "going to a safe place," "calling the police if it is safe to do so," "getting out of the way," "locking yourself in the bathroom," and "coming to The Kids' Club," among other answers. But there was disagreement as to the best approach. The children in this group learned from one another that, while not all options were considered appropriate in their own family, there are common ideas about what children can do to feel safe and that they can make safety plans.

Some poor neighborhoods and communities lack essential resources, such as shelters, whereas other poor neighborhoods are rich in social connections and supports (Ceballo & McLoyd, 2002). The availability of resources in a neighborhood can also constrain the options for the child when discussing safety planning. For example, in some neighborhoods there is little transportation, or the police do not always respond, and/or there is never an arrest of the abuser. Other researchers note that in African American families it is preferable to call family and friends rather than the police in emergencies (Williams et al., 2001). Children know from their families what is possible in their own neighborhood. Therefore, in the intervention program, group leaders need to know the local perspective, as it is fruitless and even dangerous to expect some children to call 911 for help. Further, when the program is offered to children staying in a shelter for abused women, the issues and options for safety would be expected to differ considerably.

SUMMARY AND CONCLUSIONS

In this chapter, we reviewed a number of issues pertinent to creating and implementing culturally appropriate interventions for children exposed to domestic violence. As the vignettes and studies illustrate, the various ways of surviving adversity take different pathways and are defined by different issues for children in families from diverse cultural backgrounds. We showed how cultural diversity shaped The Kids' Club program, including supervising therapists in developing cultural sensitivity, and providing culturally competent programs.

However, much of what is known about culture and clinical interventions is based on theory and clinical example. And we are still basing our practices with children on the literature developed for use with adults. Thus, much more knowledge and empirical study are needed to establish the best practices with children in this field. Many questions remain. A number of specific suggestions and recommendations for increasing our knowledge are offered below.

It is unclear whether children exposed to domestic violence are best treated in culturally similar or mixed cultural groups. Specifically, we need more studies of children in multicultural and monocultural groups so that comparisons can be made as to whether homogeneity in intervention groups provides the best experience. Similarly, a number of ethnic groups can be tested to see whether monocultural interventions are better for specific groups of children and families.

Much of what we know about intervention with children exposed to domestic violence is based on children living in shelters for abused women (Graham-Bermann, 2002). Samples of children exposed to violence in various cultural groups have to go beyond families living in shelters or departing from shelters, to those living in a range of community settings. Evaluation studies that compare the same program across settings and populations of children are most desirable and needed.

While there is a literature on the wisdom of matching the ethnicity of the therapist with the ethnicity of the adult, very little work has been done in assessing this treatment condition for work with children. Studies can be done to assess interventions from the child's viewpoint. By studying the service recipients, perhaps we can evaluate the qualities of therapists that matter to the child and the family. Similarly, to date, there is no study of the efficacy of culturally sensitive therapists versus those not trained in cultural issues when working with children. By systematically studying the service providers and the programs themselves, we can hope to identify features of programs that are particularly effective with particular groups.

Most interventions are based on a one-size-fits-all model. While this approach may be the most practical for use in communities and shelters, it is not clear whether it is best for all groups of children. Much more knowledge is needed to adequately describe the risk and protective factors that proscribe outcomes for children in various ethnic and cultural groups. To plan the most effective interventions, we need to know more about modal experiences as well as the range of experiences, and overlaps, of children in different families exposed to violence. Then, perhaps, interventions can be designed with specific goals that take relevant cultural circumstances and practices into account.

The additional challenges to adjustment posed by children in immigrant families and those new to this culture have yet to be explored. Issues particular to immigrant children, bilingual children, and bicultural children exposed to domestic violence have not been studied in detail. Perhaps we can contemplate creating interventions for children exposed to domestic violence who also have multiple traumas and/or those who are adjusting to a new culture.

Finally, we need to fund programs and studies for children exposed to domestic violence from different nationalities and ethnicities, in both the short and long term, to trace the pathways of adjustment for children in a variety of families. With a longitudinal approach, we can assess who is coping well in the face of violence and who needs help, as well as which children recover and those who get worse over time. In this way we can begin to design programs that address problems early in the life of the child to enhance adjustment and to do so in a culturally appropriate way.

REFERENCES

Allen, I. M. (1996). PTSD among African-Americans. In A. J. Marsella, M. J. Friedman, E. T. Gerrity, & R. M. Scurfield (Eds.), *Ethnocultural aspects of posttraumatic stress disorder: Issues, research, and clinical applications* (pp. 209–238). Washington, DC: American Psychological Association.

Allen, L., & Majidi-Ahi, S. (1989). Black American children. In J. T. Gibbs & L. N. Huang (Eds.), *Children of color: Psychological interventions with minority youth* (pp. 148–178). San Francisco: Jossey-Bass.

Aponte, J. F., Rivers, R. Y., & Wohl, J. (1994). *Psychological intervention with ethnically diverse groups: Concepts, issues, and methods.* Boston: Allyn & Bacon.

Bell, C. C., & Chance-Hill, G. (1991). Treatment of violent families. *Journal of the National Medical Association, 83*(3), 203–208.

Bell, C., & Mattis, J. (2000). The importance of cultural competence in ministering to African-American victims of domestic violence. *Violence Against Women, 6*(5), 515–532.

Castillo, R. (1997). *Culture and mental illness: A client-centered approach.* New York: Brooks/Cole.

Ceballo, R., & McLoyd, V. C. (2002). Social support and parenting in poor, dangerous neighborhoods. *Child Development, 73*(4), 1310–1321.

Cohler, B. J., Stott, F. M., & Musick, J. S. (1995). Adversity, vulnerability, and resilience: Cultural and developmental perspectives. In D. Cicchetti & D. J. Lynch (Eds.), *Developmental psychopathology: Vol. 2. Risk, disorder, and adaptation* (pp. 753–800). New York: Wiley.

Dana, R. H. (1993). *Multicultural Assessment Perspectives for Professional Psychology.* Needham Heights, MA: Allyn & Bacon.

Espin, O. M. (1987). Psychological impact of migration on Latinas. *Psychology of Women Quarterly, 11,* 489–503.

Garcia-Coll, C. & Magnuson, K. (1997). The psychological experience of immigration: A developmental perspective. In A. Booth, A. Crouter, & N. Landale (Eds.), *Immigration and the family: Research and policy on U.S. immigrants.* Mahwah, NJ: Erlbaum.

Gil, E. (1991). *The healing power of play: Working with abused children.* New York: Guilford Press.

Gillum, R., Gomez-Marin, O., & Prineas, R. (1984). Racial differences in personality, behavior, and family environment in Minneapolis school children. *Journal of the National Medical Association, 76,* 1097–1105.

Graham-Bermann, S. A. (1992). *The Kids' Club: A preventive intervention program for children of battered women.* University of Michigan, Department of Psychology, Ann Arbor, MI.

Graham-Bermann, S. A. (1998). The impact of woman abuse on children's social development. In G. W. Holden, R. Geffner, & E. N. Jouriles (Eds.), *Children and marital violence: Theory, research, and intervention* (pp. 21–54). Washington, DC: American Psychological Association.

Graham-Bermann, S. A. (2001). Designing intervention evaluations for children exposed to domestic violence: Applications of research and theory. In S. A. Graham-Bermann & J. L. Edleson (Eds.), *Domestic violence in the lives of children: The future of research, intervention, and social policy* (pp. 237–268). Washington, DC: American Psychological Association.

Graham-Bermann, S. A. (2002). Child abuse in the context of domestic violence. In J. E. B. Myers (Ed.), *APSAC handbook on child maltreatment* (2nd ed., pp. 119–130). Newbury Park, CA: Sage.

Graham-Bermann, S. A., & Brescoll, V. (2000). Gender, power, and violence: Assessing the family stereotypes of the children of batterers. *Journal of Family Psychology, 14*(4), 600–612.

Graham-Bermann, S. A., & Follet, C. (2000). *The Preschool Kids' Club: A preventive intervention program for children of battered women.* Department of Psychology, University of Michigan.

Graham-Bermann, S. A., & Gruber, G. (2003). *Ecological factors discriminating among resiliency and psychopathology in children of exposed to family violence.* Manuscript under review.

Graham-Bermann, S. A. & Halabu, H. (2001, June 6). *Intervention with young children exposed to family violence.* Paper presented at the Our children, our future: A call to action. An international conference on children exposed to domestic violence. London Family Court Clinic, London, Ontario.

Graham-Bermann, S. A., & Levendosky, A. A. (1994). *The moms' group: A parenting support and intervention program for battered women who are mothers.* Ann Arbor: University of Michigan.

Graham-Bermann, S. A., & Levendosky, A. A. (1998). Traumatic stress symptoms in children of battered women. *Journal of Interpersonal Violence, 14,* 111–128.

Gutierrez, L. M. (1990). Working with women of color: An empowerment perspective. *Social Work,* 149–153.

Helms, J. E. (1990). *Black and white racial identity: Theory, research, and practice.* New York: Greenwood Press.

Ho, M. K. (1992). Differential application of treatment modalities with Asian Ameican youth. In L. A. Vargas & J. D. Koss-Chioino (Eds.), *Working with culture: Psychotherapeutic interventions with ethnic minority children and adolescents* (pp. 182–203). San Francisco: Jossey-Bass.

Hokoda, A., Edleson, M. G., Tate, D., Carter, A., & Guerrero, G. (1998, October). *Moms Helping Kids (MHK): An educational program to help children cope with the effects of domestic violence.* Paper presented at the Fourth International Conference on Children Exposed to Family Violence, San Diego, CA.

Jones, A. C. (1989). Psychological functioning in African-American adults: Some elaborations on a model, with clinical applications. In R. L. Jones (Ed.) *Black adult development and aging.* Berkeley, CA: Cobb & Henry.

Kanuha, V. (1994). Women of color in battering relationships. In L. Comas-Díaz & B. Greene (Eds.), *Women of color: Integrating ethnic and gender identities in psychotherapy* (pp. 428–454). New York: Guilford Press.

Kleinman, A. (1992). How culture is important for DSM-IV. In J. E. Mezzich, A. Kleinman, H. Fabrega, B. Good, G. Johnson-Powell, K. M. Lin, S. Manson, & D. Parron (Eds.), *Cultural proposals for the DSM-IV.* DSM-IV Task Force, NIMH Group on Culture and Diagnosis. Pittsburgh, PA: University of Pittsburgh.

Masten, A. S., & Coatsworth, D. (1995). Competence, resilience, and psychopathology. In D. Cicchetti & D. Cohen (Eds.), *Developmental psychopathology: Vol. 1. Theory and methods* (pp. 715–752). New York: Wiley.

McCloskey, L. A., Figueredo, A. J., & Koss, M. P. (1995). *The effects of systemic family violence on children's mental health. Child Development, 66,* 1239–1261.

Nguyen, N. A. (1992). Living between two cultures: Treating first-generation Asian Americans. In L. A. Vargas & J. D. Koss-Chioino (Eds.), *Working with culture: Psychotherapeutic interventions with ethnic minority children and adolescents* (pp. 204–224). San Francisco, CA: Jossey-Bass.

Ogbu, J. (1990). Cultural model, identity, and literacy. In J. Stigler, R. Schweder, & G. Herdt (Eds.), *Cultural psychology: Essays on comparative human development* (pp. 520–541). New York: Cambridge University Press.

O'Keefe, M. (1994a). Racial/ethnic differences among battered women and their children. *Journal of Child and Family Studies, 3,* 283–305.

O'Keefe, M. (1994b). Adjustment of children from maritally violent homes. *Families in Society, 75*, 403–415.

Paniagua, F. A. (1998). *Assessing and treating culturally diverse clients: A practical guide* (2nd ed.). Newbury Park, CA: Sage.

Parham, T. A. (2002). *Counseling persons of African-American descent: Raising the bar of practitioner competence*. Newbury Park, CA: Sage.

Peters, M. F. (1981). Parenting in Black families with young children: A historical perspective. In H. McAdoo (Ed.), *Black families*. Newbury Park, CA: Sage.

Pope-Davis, D. B., & Coleman, H. L. K. (2001). *The intersection of race, class, and gender in multicultural counseling*. Newbury Park, CA: Sage.

Porterotto, J. G., Casas, J. M., Suzuki, L. A., & Alexander, A. M. (1995). *Handbook of multicultural counseling*. Thousand Oaks, CA: Sage.

Ramirez, O. (1989). Mexican-American children and adolescents. In. J. T. Gibbs & L. N. Huang (Eds.), *Children of color: Psychological interventions with minority youth* (pp. 223–250). San Francisco, CA: Jossey-Bass.

Roopnarine, J. L., Johnson, J. E., & Hooper, F. H. (Eds.). (1994). *Children's play in diverse cultures*. New York: SUNY Press.

Root, M. P. (1996). Women of color and traumatic stress in "domestic captivity": Gender and race as disempowering statuses. In A. J. Marsella, M. J. Friedman, E. T. Gerrity, & R. M. Scurfield (Eds.), *Ethnocultural aspects of posttraumatic stress disorder: Issues, research, and clinical applications* (pp. 363–387). Washington, DC: American Psychological Association.

Rossman, B. B. R., & Ho, J. (2000). Posttraumatic response and children exposed to parental violence. In R. A. Geffner, P. G. Jaffe, & M. Sudermann (Eds.), *Children exposed to domestic violence: Current issues in research, intervention, prevention, and policy development* (pp. 85–106). Binghamton, NY: Haworth.

Sampson, R. J. (1993). The community context of violent crime. In W. J. Wilson (Ed.), *Sociology and the Public Agency* (pp. 259–286). Newbury Park, CA: Sage.

Sluzki, C. (1979). Migration and family conflict. *Family Process, 18*(4), 379–390.

Stagg, V., Wills, G. D., & Howell, M. (1989). Psychopathology in early childhood witness of family violence, *Topics in Early Childhood Special Education, 9*, 73–87.

Suarez-Orozco, C. (2000). Identities under siege: Immigration stress and social mirroring among the children of immigrants. In A. C. G. M. Robben & M. M. Suarez-Orozco (Eds.), *Cultures under siege: Collective violence and trauma* (pp. 194–226). London: Cambridge University Press.

Sue, S. (1988). Psychotherapeutic service for ethnic minorities: Two decades of research findings. *American Psychologist, 43*(4), 301–308.

Sue, S. (1998). In search of cultural competence in psychotherapy and counseling. *American Psychologist, 53*(4), 440–448.

Tseng, W. S., & Hsu, J. (1980). Minor psychological disturbances of everyday life. In H. Triandis & J. G. Draguns (Eds.), *Handbook of cross-cultural psychology: Vol. 1. Psychopathology* (pp. 61–97). Boston: Allyn & Bacon.

U.S. Surgeon General. (2001). *Mental health: Culture, race and ethnicity.* A supplement to Mental Health: A Report of the Surgeon General. Rockville, MD: U.S. Department of Health and Human Services (S. Lopez, S. Manson, J. Miranda, L. Snowden, & S. Sue, Science Editors).

Weisz, J. R., Suwanlert, S., Chaiyasit, W., Weiss, B., Achenbach, T., & Eastman, K. L. (1993). Behavioral and emotional problems among Thai and American adolescents: Parent reports for ages 12–16. *Journal of Abnormal Psychology, 102,* 395–403.

Westra, B., & Martin, H. P. (1981). Children of battered women. *Maternal Child Nursing, 10,* 41–54.

Williams, O., Boggess, J. L., & Carter, J. (2001). Fatherhood and domestic violence: Exploring the role of men who batter in the lives of their children. In S. A. Graham-Bermann & J. L. Edleson (Eds.), *Domestic violence in the lives of children: The future of research, intervention, and social policy* (pp. 283–298). Washington, DC: American Psychological Association.

Willis, D. J., Dobrec, A., & Sipes, D. S. B. F. (1992). Treating American Indian victims of abuse and neglect. In L. A. Vargas & J. D. Koss-Chioino (Eds.), *Working with culture: Psychotherapeutic interventions with ethnic minority children and adolescents* (pp. 276–299). San Francisco, CA: Jossey-Bass.

Zane, H., Hall, G. N., Sue, S., Young, K., & Nunez, J. (2002). Research on psychotherapy with culturally diverse populations. In M. J. Lambert, A. E. Bergin, & S. L. Garfield (Eds.), *Handbook of psychotherapy and behavior change* (5th ed.). New York: Wiley.

6

Safety Planning for Abused Women and Their Children

JENNIFER L. HARDESTY and JACQUELYN C. CAMPBELL

Safety planning has become the most frequently mentioned intervention for abused women in both advocacy and professional literature and training. Yet, what is meant by safety planning is seldom completely described. There are many published prescriptions for safety planning, including many detailed tools meant to be filled out by abused women with or without the help of an advocate. These forms vary widely in their content and length, and there have been no published evaluations of the efficacy of safety planning. Even so, most advocates and professionals agree that safety planning is an important component of intervention in cases of domestic violence. Generally, the purpose is to work with the woman to identify how she can act to better keep herself safe from further acts of intimate partner violence. In this way, the plan is context- and case-specific and helps increase what has been identified as the woman's own agency, or ability to take care of herself (Campbell & Soeken, 1999; Lempert, 1996).

Traditionally, however, safety plans have not accounted for mothering concerns and safety strategies for children after separation. Abused women are usually good mothers dedicated to nurturing and protecting their children (Humphreys, 1995; Sullivan, Nguyen, Allen, Bybee, & Juras, 2000). Their decision to leave an abusive partner is influenced greatly by concerns for their children. After leaving, they want to make decisions in the best interests of their children (Ericksen & Henderson, 1998; Henderson, 1990; Humphreys, 1993). Many face the dilemma of balancing their own and their children's need for safety with their belief that children need an ongoing relationship with their father (Hardesty & Ganong, 2003). They may compromise their own safety to ensure the latter, believing that continued father contact is best for their children. Others are required by courts to maintain contact through shared parenting arrangements (Jaffe & Geffner, 1998). Either way, abused mothers are likely to have continued exposure to their abusers after separation, and abusers may continue to control and abuse them through these parenting arrangements (Hardesty & Ganong, 2003). Thus, post-separation safety planning specific to women who share children with their abusers is needed.

SAFETY PLANNING BASED ON LETHALITY ASSESSMENT

One of the crucial bases of safety planning is an accurate and detailed assessment of the degree of danger that the woman is experiencing. Several risk factor lists and instruments have been developed over the past few years, including the Danger Assessment (DA) (Campbell, 1995; Campbell, Sharps, & Glass, 2000). This instrument is a short (17-item) yes/no risk factor list designed to help women assess their own risk of homicide or serious abuse from a violent relationship. Although many advocates stress that women are the best judge of their amount of risk, in a recent study of risk factors for intimate partner femicide, approximately half of both actual and attempted femicide victims did not think their partner was capable of killing them (Campbell et al., in press). Therefore, although women's assessment of their own danger should always be one of the factors assessed, they also may need help in accurately identifying the pattern of abuse and other risk factors. The DA therefore starts with a calendar assessment, where the woman first marks on a calendar (computer-generated) of the past year the dates and severity of each abusive incident. Using a calendar increases recall in many contexts (Belli, Shay, & Stafford, 2001). This domestic violence specific calendar gives the woman and the practitioner helping with safety planning an accurate picture of the pattern of violence, including escalation of severity and/or frequency, if that is occurring.

In recent DA validation work (Campbell et al., in press), the DA has been slightly modified (see Figure 6.1). This reflects the serious risks found related to threats to the children as well as the woman having another partner. In addition, other risk factors for femicide include abuse during pregnancy and the presence of a stepchild in the home (a biological child of the mother but not the abuser) (see also Daly, Wiseman, & Wilson, 1997). All of the risk factors on the original DA were found to be associated with significantly more risk of femicide or attempted femicide except for the woman's suicidality. However, an abused woman's potential suicide is an important issue of danger and one that should be assessed regardless. It also may be a risk factor for the woman killing her abusive partner (Campbell, 1995) and for those two reasons, it remained a factor on the DA.

There is not yet any "cutoff" score on the DA—the more yeses, the more risk. The higher the score, the more assertive the practitioner should be in safety planning, keeping in mind that in prior studies scores of 8 or more were found in the groups at the highest risk (Campbell et al., 2000; Campbell et al., in press). By looking at the score, the woman sees for herself the amount of danger. This "reality check" is an important beginning to subsequent safety planning. When the woman says she has left the abuser or is planning to leave the abuser, the recent femicide study as well as prior research (Campbell et al., in press) suggests even higher degrees of risk. Thus, the woman should be urged to not tell her abuser face-to-face she is leaving. It is very important that she leave with the children at a time he is not present and then call from a place unknown to him (preferably a shelter) to tell him she has left and discuss ongoing issues with the children. This discussion with him is very important in terms of the woman gauging future risk, especially if he makes threats of harming her or the children or of killing himself. Homicide–suicide cases make up approximately one-third of intimate partner femicides, and children may be the other victims in these cases (Websdale, 1999).

SAFETY PLANNING FOR SPECIFIC CHILD-RELATED ISSUES

Although not all separations or divorces involve child access or custody disputes, abusive men may be more likely to fight for custody than nonabusive men (Zorza, 1995). Also many couples in high-conflict divorces approach legal professionals seeking alternatives to legal disputes,

FIGURE 6.1. Danger Assessment. Jacquelyn C. Campbell, PhD, RN. Copyright 1985, 1988, 2001.

Several risk factors have been associated with homicides (murders) of both batterers and battered women in research conducted after the murders have taken place. We cannot predict what will happen in your case, but we would like you to be aware of the danger of homicide in situations of severe battering and for you to see how many of the risk factors apply to your situation. Using the calendar, please mark the approximate dates during the past year when you were beaten by your husband or partner. Write on that date how bad the incident was according to the following scale:

1. Slapping, pushing; no injuries and/or lasting pain
2. Punching, kicking; bruises, cuts, and/or continuing pain
3. "Beating up"; severe contusions, burns, broken bones
4. Threat to use weapon; head injury, internal injury, permanent injury
5. Use of weapon; wounds from weapon

(If **any** of the descriptions for the higher number apply, use the higher number.)
Mark **Yes** or **No** for each of the following. ("He" refers to your husband, partner, ex-husband, ex-partner, or whoever is currently physically hurting you.)

_____ 1. Has the physical violence increased in severity or frequency over the past year?
_____ 2. Has he ever used a weapon or threatened you with a weapon?
_____ 3. Does he ever try to choke you?
_____ 4. Does he have access to a gun?
_____ 5. Has he ever forced you to have sex when you did not wish to do so?
_____ 6. Does he use drugs? By drugs, I mean "uppers" or amphetamines, speed, angel dust, cocaine, "crack," street drugs, or mixtures.
_____ 7. Does he threaten to kill you and/or do you believe he is capable of killing you?
_____ 8. Is he drunk every day or almost every day (in terms of quantity of alcohol)?
_____ 9. Does he control most or all of your daily activities? For instance: does he tell you who you can be friends with, when you can see your family, how much money you can use, or when you can take the car? (If he tries, but you do not let him, check here: _____.)
_____ 10. Have you ever been beaten by him while you were pregnant? (If you have never been pregnant by him, check here: _____.)
_____ 11. Is he violently and constantly jealous of you? (For instance, does he say, "If I can't have you, no one can"?)
_____ 12. Have you ever threatened or tried to commit suicide?
_____ 13. Has he ever threatened or tried to commit suicide?
_____ 14. Does he threaten to harm your children?
_____ 15. Do you have a child that is not his?
_____ 16. Is he unemployed?
_____ 17. Have you left him during the past year? (If you have *never* lived with him, check here: _____.)
_____ 18. Do you currently have another (different) intimate partner?
_____ 19. Does he follow or spy on you, leave threatening notes, destroy your property, or call you when you don't want him to?

_____ Total "Yes" answers

Thank you.
Please talk to your nurse, advocate, or counselor about what the Danger Assessment means in terms of your situation.

and some of these couples have a history of domestic violence (Jaffe, Poisson, & Cunningham, 2001). Thus, a considerable number of custody disputes may involve parents with a history of domestic violence. Ensuring women's safety during custody negotiations is essential, considering the increased risk of abuse during and after separation.

As discussed in detail in Chapters 11 and 12, most states have implemented laws to protect abused women during custody negotiations (e.g., presumptions against granting joint or sole custody to spousal abusers) and to provide them with options for safe postseparation parenting arrangements (e.g., supervised visitation centers; Bartlett, 2000; Family Violence Project, 1995). Nonetheless, many abused women in the legal system remain unrecognized and uninformed about what options are available to them. To ensure their safety, courts must identify abused women in the legal system. One necessary step is to develop protocols to routinely screen for domestic violence in child custody cases.

If initial screening indicates abuse, several steps can be taken to prioritize safety during negotiations. A legal professional or advocate should work with the woman to first assess her degree of risk, using the DA. Her level of risk should then inform the court's decisions during negotiations. For example, if there is indication of moderate or high risk, mediation or face-to-face negotiations should be avoided. Steps can also be taken to ensure the woman's safety if she must be present with the abuser in court or if she must attend any court-mandated programs (e.g., classes for divorcing parents). The abuser and victim should attend such programs separately, and the time and date of the woman's attendance should be kept confidential. A legal professional or advocate should also work with the woman to develop an individualized parenting plan based on the history of abuse, the level of risk to her, and the individual needs of the parties involved. Specific provisions for safety should be included in the plan (see Table 6.1). The woman should be informed about the different legal options (e.g., mandating batterers intervention as a condition of visitation) and community services (e.g., visitation centers) available to her so that she can develop a parenting plan that prioritizes safety.

A legal professional or advocate can help the woman identify potential risks involved in various shared parenting options. For example, a key risk factor is the abuser's access to the victim, making unsupervised visitations and exchanges a risky time for severe or lethal violence to the victim or harm to the children (Sheeran & Hampton, 1999). Also, joint custody arrangements, usually assumed to be in the best interests of children, may not be warranted in cases with woman abuse (Jaffe et al., 2001). Visitation and custody should be awarded only when adequate provision for safety of the victim and children can be assured (Family Vi-

TABLE 6.1. Recommendations for a Safety-Focused Parenting Plan

To the degree necessary to ensure safety, parenting plans should specify:

- Days and times of visits and exact times for exchanges.
- Who will supervise visits if supervised visitation is ordered (e.g., neutral third party, trained professional, family member, visitation center personnel).
- Where the children will be exchanged (e.g., public setting, in the presence of a third party, through a third party).
- How the children will be exchanged (e.g., father must drop off children with third party and leave the exchange location before the mother arrives).
- How issues related to the children will be discussed (e.g., in person, on the telephone, via written communications only).
- How child support will be provided and how issues related to child support will be discussed (e.g., children will not be asked to relay messages about money).
- Any prohibitions related to the father's drug and alcohol consumption before or during visits.
- Any requirements the father must meet in order to continue visits (e.g., complete counseling, batterer intervention program, substance abuse treatment, parenting classes).
- Any prohibitions related to traveling with children during visits (e.g., no out-of-state travel).
- Any prohibitions related to weapons (e.g., removal of firearms during visits).
- Under what circumstances arrangements can be denied or canceled (e.g., sick child, father intoxicated).
- What to do if a visit is missed (e.g., substitute another day).
- What to do if any conditions of the parenting plan are violated (e.g., visits suspended if abuse occurs, child returns to mother's home if he or she feels afraid, return to court to modify parenting plan).
- What rights the children have during visits (e.g., to contact their mother during visits, to not be interrogated about their mother, to terminate the visit at any time).
- What to do if the parenting plan needs modification because of children's changing needs or because circumstances change (e.g., return to court for legal modification, informal agreements acceptable).

Note. Suggestions based on the authors' work and Hart (2001).

olence Project, 1995). A court-approved parenting plan that includes specific and detailed agreements (see Table 6.2) offers an additional element of protection if the perpetrator violates the order.

To help women prioritize safety, legal professionals and advocates would benefit from acknowledging the context within which abused women make decisions about postseparation parenting. There is much attention to options available for women who wish to restrict the abuser's access to them and their children (e.g., protection orders, supervised visitation). As explored in Chapter 7, less is known about what options are available to women who want to share parenting with their children's father, or women who wish to facilitate father–child contact provided that their own contact with their former partner is limited. Many abused women want their children to maintain a relationship with their father (Hardesty & Ganong, 2003). Despite a history of abuse, they believe he is a good father. Such views are not surprising, considering societal values emphasizing that children fare better in two-parent families than in divorced families. Women may feel guilty about "breaking up" a two-parent family, or they may believe that denying father–child contact is harmful to children. Legal professionals and advocates should acknowledge this dilemma and help abused women consider shared parenting options that balance continued contact with safety.

Finally, legal professionals and advocates should encourage abused women to consider long-term safety needs when developing parenting plans. For example, specific guidelines for modifying the parenting plan to meet the developing needs of children over time can be included in the original document. Abused women have expressed the need for plans to protect their children, both in immediate situations and in the future (Humphreys, 1995). In one study, women who were co-parenting indicated ongoing efforts to set limits and boundaries with their abusive former husband to ensure their safety over time (Hardesty & Ganong, 2003). Abused women would benefit from "anticipatory guidance" (Henderson, 1990, p. 13), or parenting preparation that helps women anticipate problems associated with ongoing contact. For example, guidance on setting limits with former partners and enforcing the parenting plan would be useful. To ensure ongoing safety, subsequent assessments of risk are needed any time a woman returns to court to modify the parenting plan.

SAFETY PLANNING FOR CHILDREN

Supporting and ensuring the safety of abused mothers is one effective way to ensure the safety of children (Radford & Hester, 2001). Traditionally, however, children have not been a part of the safety planning process. Children need specific safety planning strategies, especially during the high-risk time after separation when they are likely to have unsupervised contact with their fathers.

The purpose of safety planning is to empower children to identify safety issues and problem solve in ways that will protect themselves (Hart, 2001). Hart (2001) suggests that a professional should facilitate safety planning with the child so that the mother does not appear "hostile" toward the father during custody negotiations. To appreciate the mother's concern for her child, however, the practitioner should involve her in the process. Specific safety strategies related to the children can also be included in the parenting plan (see Table 6.1). As with their mother's, safety planning should be informed by an assessment of danger and lethality.

Safety planning will be most helpful to children if practitioners and mothers recognize the individual needs of the children. Practitioners need to assess with the mother the following characteristics of the children before tailoring with her an individualized safety plan: (1) age/developmental status; (2) mental status; (3) physical health status; and (4) attachment to the father (e.g., the degree of ambivalence or conflicted feelings toward the father). More specifically, safety plans must be age-appropriate, and the child must be capable of and competent enough to carry them out. Development also should be considered both in terms of understanding and responding to violence. For example, in planning for what to do during visits if things get dangerous, an older child may be more able to dial 911 whereas it may be safer to instruct a younger child to go to the neighbors. Also, it may be more necessary with older children to advise them to escape and not try to intervene than with younger children who are less likely to intervene. It is also necessary to take into account the degree of attachment the child has to the abuser. For instance, it may be unreasonable to expect a boy strongly attached to his father to call the police on his "dad." Safety planning is necessary to minimize risk, but it also can help reduce children's anxiety and fears about unsupervised visits (Hart, 2001).

Practitioners can also assess the availability of social supports to assist children in safety planning. Children need support systems other than their mother, especially if they are having difficulty dealing with their parents' separation or if they feel loyalty conflicts between their parents. A child may feel ambivalent toward the mother and her decision to leave the father. The child might blame the mother for not being able to see the father as often as before. Outside sources of support can provide valuable opportunities for children to share their conflicting feelings and avoid getting "caught in the middle" by confiding in a parent. Practitioners can encourage the mother to elicit support from formal or informal support systems to provide her child with a caring adult to talk to. A caring and trusted adult also can provide the child with a safe place to go when necessary.

One source of support is within the school system (e.g., teacher, principal, school nurse, counselor). Mothers usually feel safe with their children at school (some feel unsafe leaving children without their supervision). School personnel can serve as a confidante for the child, and they can alert the mother to signs of significant problems (e.g., behavioral or academic problems). The mother can keep the school informed of specific custody arrangements (e.g., who has permission to pick the child up from school) and any changes or problems that occur. Being aware of potential stressors for the child (e.g., adjusting to a new visitation schedule) can help teachers understand and manage any changes in the child's behavior or performance in school. A limitation to involving school personnel is that they may not be adequately trained to respond to issues of domestic violence, or they may feel that providing such support is not part of their role. As mandated reporters, they may violate the child's trust if they must report information the child discloses to them. As discussed further in Chapter 13, training school personnel about the dynamics of divorce and domestic violence and ways that they can provide support to parents and children would be beneficial.

Another source of support is the health care system. Again, there are pros and cons in involving health care clinicians. Health care providers are mandated reporters of child abuse, and in states where witnessing domestic violence is child abuse, they would be mandated reporters of this form of abuse. However, except in those states and in cases where child abuse is occurring, health care providers will keep information about domestic violence in the home confidential. It is important for the child's health care provider to know about domestic violence between the parents in order to make fully informed diagnoses and treatment decisions about a wide variety of the children's health care problems. There is evidence that such physical health conditions as enuresis (bedwetting) and asthma exacerbation may be related to the stress of witnessing domestic violence (Kernic et al., 2002). Episodes of these kinds of problems may be noted as occurring before and/or after visitations with the father or various legal proceedings. Health care providers need to plan with mothers and the children about how to anticipate and manage these symptoms.

Children who witness domestic violence also have been shown to have more communicable diseases and miss more time from school than other children, perhaps because of a compromised immune system due to high stress levels (Campbell & Parker, 2000; Hurt, Malmud, Brodsky, & Giannetta, 2001; Kerouac, Taggart, Lescop, & Fortin, 1986). Even more serious long-term physical health problems have been identified for children who are victims of child abuse (Kernic et al., 2002). Since witnessing domestic violence and child abuse victimization are significantly likely to co-occur, many of the children of abused women will have an increase in physical health problems related to these effects. The state of the science in regard to physical health effects of children witnessing intimate partner violence with or without concurrent child abuse is based on only a few investigations. No doubt there are other physical health effects for children witnessing domestic violence that have yet to be identified, just because they have not been studied. Therefore, to provide the

TABLE 6.2. Categories of Assessment for Battered Women with Children

- Danger Assessment
  - Degree of risk to women
  - Degree of risk to children—for child abuse, for lethality
- Age/developmental status of children
- Mental status of children
- Physical health status of children
- Attachment to perpetrator

best health care for their children, mothers and domestic violence advocates should generally make health care providers an informed part of the team that is addressing the welfare of their children. Only by knowing about the prior domestic violence in the home and the potential ongoing stressors related to the father, including visitation and custody issues, can the health care provider take into account this form of stress in addressing the children's welfare.

SUMMARY AND CONCLUSIONS

Safety planning for abused women with children is needed, as these women are likely to have ongoing contact with their abusers after the relationship ends. Safety planning should empower women and build on their abilities as mothers. Legal professionals and domestic violence advocates can enlist and invest in women based on their concerns for their children and assist them in prioritizing safety in custody negotiations. The varieties of contingencies that need to be taken into account make it very difficult to formulate a tool for safety planning that can be used in all situations. Rather, there needs to be a format for assessing each of the different categories of concern and then developing plans based on those assessments. Safety assessment strategies have been suggested throughout this chapter and are summarized in Table 6.2.

REFERENCES

Bartlett, K. T. (2000). Improving the law relating to postdivorce arrangements for children. In R. A. Thompson & P. R. Amato (Eds.), *The postdivorce family: Children, parenting, and society* (pp. 71–102). Thousand Oaks, CA: Sage.

Belli, R. F., Shay, W. L., & Stafford, F. P. (2001). Event history calendars and question list surveys: A direct comparison of interviewing methods. *Public opinion quarterly, 65,* 45–74.

Campbell, J. C. (1995). *Assessing dangerousness.* Newbury Park, CA: Sage.

Campbell, J. C., Koziol-McLain, J., Glass, N. E., Webster, D., Block, R., McFarlane, J., & Campbell, D. W. (in press). *Validation of the danger assessment: Results from the 12 city femicide study.* National Institute of Justice Briefs.

Campbell, J. C., & Parker, B. (1999). Clinical nursing research on battered women and their children. In A. S. Hinshaw, S. L. Feetham, & J. L. F. Shaver (Eds.), *Handbook of clinical nursing research* (pp. 535–559). Thousand Oaks, CA: Sage.

Campbell, J. C., Sharps, P. W., & Glass, N. E. (2000). Risk assessment for intimate partner homicide. In G. F. Pinard & L. Pagani (Eds.), *Clinical assessment of dangerousness: Empirical contributions* (pp. 136–157). New York: Cambridge University Press.

Campbell, J. C., & Soeken, K. L. (1999). Women's responses to battering: A test of the model. *Research in Nursing and Health,* 22(1), 49–58.

Daly, M., Wiseman, K. A., & Wilson, M. (1997). Women and children sired by previous partners incur excess risk of uxoricide. *Homicide Studies, 1*(1), 61–71.

Ericksen, J. R., & Henderson, A. D. (1998). Diverging realities: Abused women and their children. In J. C. Campbell (Ed.), *Empowering survivors of abuse: Health care for battered women and their children* (pp. 138–155). Thousand Oaks, CA: Sage.

Family Violence Project of The National Council of Juvenile and Family Court Judges. (1995). Family violence in child custody statutes: An analysis of state codes and legal practice. *Family Law Quarterly, 29,* 195–225.

Ford Gilboe, M. (1997). Family strengths, motivation and resources as predictors of health promotion behaviour in single-parent families. *Research in Nursing and Health, 20*(3) 205–217.

Ford-Gilboe, M. (2001). Making connections: A vehicle for developing a nursing response to violence against women and children in Canada. *Canadian Journal of Nursing Research, 32*(4), 125–134.

Hardesty, J. L., & Ganong, L. H. (2003). *A grounded theory model of negotiating custody and post-divorce parenting with an abusive former husband.* Manuscript under review.

Hart, B. J. (2001). Safety planning for children: Strategizing for unsupervised visits with batterers. *Minnesota Center Against Violence and Abuse.* Retrieved from *http://www.mincava.umn.edu/hart/safetyp.htm.*

Henderson, A. (1990, June/September). Children of abused wives: Their influence on their mothers' decisions. *Canada's Mental Health, 38,* 10–13.

Humphreys, J. (1993). Helping battered women care for their children. In J. C. Campbell (Ed.), *AWHONN's clinical issues in perinatal and women's health nursing: Domestic violence, 4*(3) (pp. 458–470). Philadelphia: Lippincott.

Humphreys, J. (1995). The work of worrying: Battered women and their children. *Scholarly Inquiry for Nursing Practice: An International Journal, 9*(2), 127–145.

Hurt, H., Malmud, E., Brodsky, N. L., & Giannetta, J. (2001). Exposure to violence: Psychological and academic correlates in child witnesses. *Archives of
Pediatric and Adolescent Medicine, 155*(12), 1351–1356.

Jaffe, P. G., & Geffner, R. (1998). Child custody disputes and domestic violence:
Critical issues for mental health, social service, and legal professionals. In
G. W. Holden, R. Geffner, & E. N. Jouriles (Eds.), *Children exposed to
marital violence: Theory, research, and applied issues* (pp. 371–408). Washington, DC: American Psychological Association.

Jaffe, P. G., Poisson, S. E., & Cunningham, A. (2001). Domestic violence and
high-conflict divorce: Developing a new generation of research for children.
In S. A. Graham-Bermann & J. L. Edleson (Eds.), *Domestic violence in the
lives of children: The future of research, intervention, and social policy* (pp.
189–202). Washington, DC: American Psychological Association.

Kernic, M. A., Holt, V. L., Wolf, M. E., McKnight, B., Huebner, C. E., & Rivara,
F. P. (2002). Academic and school health issues among children exposed to
maternal intimate partner abuse. *Archives of Pediatric and Adolescent
Medicine, 156*(6), 549–555.

Kerouac, S., Taggart, M. E., Lescop, J., & Fortin, M. F. (1986). Dimensions of
health in violent families. *Health Care for Women International, 7,* 413–
426.

Lempert, L. B. (1996). Women's strategies for survival: Developing agency in
abusive relationships. *Journal of Family Violence, 11,* 269–290.

Radford, L., & Hester, M. (2001). Overcoming mother blaming?: Future direc-
tions for research on mothering and domestic violence. In S. A. Graham-
Bermann & J. L. Edleson (Eds.), *Domestic violence in the lives of children:
The future of research, intervention, and social policy* (pp. 135–155).
Washington DC: American Psychological Association.

Sheeran, M., & Hampton, S. (1999, Spring). Supervised visitation in cases of domestic violence. *Juvenile and Family Court Journal, 50*(2), 13–26.

Sullivan, C. M., Nguyen, H., Allen, N., Bybee, D., & Juras, J. (2000). Beyond
searching for deficits: Evidence that physically and emotionally abused
women are nurturing parents. *Journal of Emotional Abuse, 2*(1), 51–71.

Websdale, N. (1999). *Understanding domestic homicide.* Boston: Northeastern
University Press.

Zorza, J. (1995). How abused women can use the law to help protect their children. In E. Peled, P. Jaffe, & J. Edleson (Eds.), *Ending the cycle of violence:
Community responses to children of battered women* (pp. 147–169). Thousand Oaks, CA: Sage.

7

Assessing Abusers' Risks to Children

LUNDY BANCROFT and JAY G. SILVERMAN

The mounting social and professional awareness of the negative effects on children of exposure to domestic violence has drawn attention to the need for effective tools for assessing risk to children from abusers as parents or guardians (e.g., Williams, Boggess, & Carter, 2001). Such tools are particularly needed by child protective personnel, custody evaluators, and courts with jurisdiction over child custody and child welfare cases, but are also important to the work of many therapists, abused women's service providers, batterer intervention programs, and programs for children exposed to domestic violence.

The model we are proposing in this chapter is particularly suited to assessment of postseparation risk to children from abusers. We commonly encounter the mistaken assumption among professionals, including judges and custody evaluators, that children are in less danger from an abuser once a couple is no longer living together, when the reality is often the opposite (Bancroft & Silverman, 2002; Langford, Isaac, & Kabat, 1999). Assessment of risk to children postseparation should be carried out with as much caution as would be called for in intervening with an intact family.

While couples are still living together, an abuser's danger to children can be mediated to some extent by their mother's ability to protect them. Elements such as the level of physical dangerousness of the perpetrator, the mother's strengths as a parent, the ability of her community to provide the necessary legal and supportive resources, and the mother's capacity to seek and use help for herself and her children must be examined to assess her ability to protect (Whitney & Davis, 1999), while also avoiding the mistake of characterizing an abused woman as "failing to protect" her children (Magen, 1999). Therefore, the use of our model in assessing risk in intact families needs to be combined with careful and compassionate assessment of the mother's protective capabilities and her willingness to work collaboratively with child protective personnel.

RISKS TO CHILDREN POSTSEPARATION

Risk of Exposure to Threats or Acts of Violence Toward Their Mother

As mentioned in Chapter 6, a high rate of serious assaults by abusers occurs postseparation (Tjaden and Thoennes, 2000), and children are likely to witness these incidents (Peled, 2000). The risk that the perpetrator will assault the mother sexually also increases during and after separation (review in Mahoney & Williams, 1998). When an abuser kills his former partner, children commonly witness the homicide or its aftermath, or are murdered themselves (Langford et al., 1999). Many perpetrators of domestic violence homicides have little or no criminal record involving violence (Langford et al., 1999; Websdale, 1999), complicating the assessment process. Exposure to postseparation threats or assaults on the mother can also impede children's emotional healing.

Risk of Undermining Mother–Child Relationships

Abusive behavior can undermine mother–child relationships and maternal authority in a wide array of ways (Radford & Hester, 2001; McGee, 2000; Hughes & Marshall, 1995), interference which tends to continue or increase postseparation (Bancroft & Silverman, 2002). The emotional recovery of children who have been exposed to domestic violence appears to depend on the quality of their relationship with the nonabusive parent more than on any other single factor (see below), and thus perpetrators who create tensions between mothers and children can sabotage the healing process.

Risk of Physical or Sexual Abuse of the Child by the Abuser

As explored in Chapter 2, multiple studies have demonstrated the dramatically elevated rate of child physical abuse (review in McGee, 2000) and child sexual abuse (e.g. McCloskey, Figueredo, & Koss, 1995; Sirles & Franke, 1989; Paveza, 1988) by abusers. This risk may increase postseparation from the mother's inability to monitor the abuser's parenting and from the retaliatory tendencies of many abusers.

Risk to Children of the Abuser as a Role Model

Sons of abusers have dramatically elevated rates of domestic violence perpetration when they reach adulthood (Silverman & Williamson, 1997; Straus, 1990), and daughters of abusers find it more difficult than other women to seek assistance if they are abused (Doyne et al., 1999).

Risk of Rigid, Authoritarian Parenting

Recovery in traumatized children is best facilitated by a nurturing, loving environment that also includes appropriate structure, limits, and predictability. A perpetrator may be severely controlling toward children (McGee, 2000), and is likely to use a harsh, rigid disciplinary style (Margolin, John, Ghosh, & Gordis, 1996; Holden & Ritchie, 1991) that can intimidate children who have been exposed to his violence. This style can cause the reawakening of traumatic memories, setting back postseparation healing.

Risk of Neglectful or Irresponsible Parenting

Abusers often have difficulty focusing on their children's needs, due to their selfish and self-centered tendencies (Jacobson & Gottman, 1998). In postseparation visitation situations, these parenting weaknesses can be accentuated, as abusers may be caring for children for much longer periods of time than they are accustomed to. Additionally, many of our abusive clients have used intentionally neglectful parenting as a way to win their children's loyalty, for example, by not imposing appropriate safety or eating guidelines, or by permitting the children to watch inappropriate violence or sexuality in media. Neglectful parenting in our clients commonly takes the form of intermittently showing interest in their children and then ignoring them for extended periods. Postseparation, abusers with this parenting style tend to drop in and out of visitation, which can be emotionally injurious to their children and disruptive to life in the custodial home.

Risk of Psychological Abuse and Manipulation

Perpetrators tend toward verbally abusive parenting styles (McGee, 2000; Adams, 1991) and using the children as weapons against the mother (McGee, 2000; Erickson & Henderson, 1998; Peled, 1998). The latter risk appears to increase postseparation (McMahon & Pence, 1995), with visitation becoming an opportunity for an abuser to manipulate the children in his continuing efforts to control their mother (Erickson & Henderson, 1998).

Risk of Abduction

A majority of parental abductions take place in the context of domestic violence, and are mostly carried out by abusers or their agents (Greif & Hegar, 1993). Postseparation parental abductions happen most commonly 2 or more years subsequent to the separation, and about half occur during an authorized visit (Finkelhor, Hotaling, & Sedlak, 1990).

Risk of Exposure to Violence in Their Father's New Relationships

Postseparation, children run the risk that their father will abuse a new partner, as it is common for perpetrators to abuse women serially (Dutton, 1995; Woffordt, Mihalic, & Menard, 1994).

CHILDREN'S RECOVERY FROM EXPOSURE TO DOMESTIC VIOLENCE

When an abuser is no longer present in the children's home, the possibility exists that healing and recovery will begin, as demonstrated by many studies on children's resilience (review in Wolak & Finkelhor, 1998). However, we find that children's continued contact with the abuser sometimes interferes with the creation of a healing context. A number of critical elements contribute to the creation of this context.

A Sense of Physical and Emotional Safety in Their Current Surroundings

The establishment of safety, and of the feeling of safety, is a first and indispensable step toward any process of emotional healing from trauma (van der Kolk & McFarlane, 1996), and in particular for children whose experience has included fear, danger, and insecurity at home as tends to be true of children of abused women (McGee, 2000). When children are aware of the perpetrator's capacity for violence, unsupervised contact with him may cause them to feel insecure or anxious.

Structure, Limits, and Predictability

Domestic violence can create a sense of chaos and lack of predictability in the children's environment. The parenting patterns that accompany domestic violence can aggravate this problem, as abusers tend to alternate between harshness and leniency with children (Holden & Ritchie, 1991) and abused mothers often experience erosion of their authority (Hughes & Marshall, 1995). Children's healing therefore depends on the development of structure, limits, and predictability in their home life to counteract the previous experiences of fear and turmoil.

A Strong Bond to the Nonabusing Parent

Children who have experienced profound emotional distress or trauma are largely dependent for their recovery on the quality of their relationship with their caregiving parent (Jaffe & Geffner, 1998; reviews in Heller, Larrieu, D'Imperio, & Boris, 1998, and Graham-Bermann, 1998). Assisting abused mothers and their children in healing their relationships is one of the most important aspects of promoting recovery (Erickson & Henderson, 1998). Progress toward this goal may be eroded if the perpetrator uses visitation as a time to encourage the children to disrespect their mother, to feel ashamed of being close to her, or to defy her authority.

Not to Feel Responsible to Take Care of Adults

Children who are exposed to domestic violence may believe that they must protect their mother, father, or siblings. To relieve this stress, adults need to avoid burdening the children with adult concerns. The self-centeredness common in abusers leads to a substantial risk that the father may demand emotional caretaking from his children, particularly in the painful aftermath of parental separation.

A Strong Bond to Their Siblings

Overall level of family support is important in fostering resilience (Heller et al., 1998). Children exposed to domestic violence often have unusually high levels of tension in their sibling relationships (Hurley & Jaffe, 1990) and may need assistance in addressing the divisions that have occurred.

Abusers often foment tensions between siblings through favoritism and other tactics (Bancroft & Silverman, 2002), undercutting their recovery.

Contact with the Abusive Parent with Strong Protection for Children's Physical and Emotional Safety

Except in those cases involving the most terrifying abusers or those who have abused the children physically or sexually, children's recovery may be furthered by having an ongoing opportunity to express their love for their father, to have a sense that he knows them, and to be able to tell him about key events in their lives. They may also crave reassurance that he is not in overwhelming distress. However, such contact is counterproductive when it interferes with the creation of a healing context.

ASSESSING RISK TO CHILDREN FROM CONTACT WITH ABUSERS

Given the range of sources of psychological and physical injury to children from abusers and the many elements necessary for children's recovery, assessing risk to children from abusers is a complex process. Information about a perpetrator's history of behavior and attitudes has to be gathered from multiple sources, as his own reporting is not likely to be reliable (Adams, 1991; Follingstad, Rutledge, Berg, Hause, & Polek, 1990). Sources should include the mother, the children, past partners of the abuser, court and police records, child protective records, medical records, school personnel, and anyone who has witnessed relevant events. (Custody evaluators have not typically considered this type of investigating and fact gathering important to their assessments—see Bow & Quinnell, 2001). The facts gathered should then be applied in evaluating each of the following 13 points:

1. *Level of physical danger to the mother.* The higher the severity or frequency of an abuser's level of violence, the greater the risk that he will physically abuse children (Straus, 1990). Level of violence is also an indicator of a perpetrator's likelihood of attempting to kill the mother (Websdale, 1999; Langford et al., 1999) or to carry out other continued assaults against her (Weisz, Tolman, & Saunders, 2000). His history of sexually assaulting the mother is correlated to overall level of physical danger (Campbell, Soeken, McFarlane, & Parker, 1998) and specifically to his likelihood of physically abusing children (Bowker, Arbitell, & McFerron, 1988). Threats of abuse are highly correlated with future physical violence (Follingstad et al., 1990), including postseparation vio-

lence (Fleury, Sullivan, & Bybee, 2000). Evaluators should note that both threatened and actual homicide attempts may take place in cases where the abuser's previous history of violence had not been severe (McCloskey et al., 1995), and that the woman's own assessment of the likelihood of future violence by an abuser may be more accurate than any other predictor (Weisz et al., 2000).

Additional relevant questions include: Has the perpetrator ever choked the mother? What types of injuries has he caused? Has he ever violated a restraining order? Has he made death threats against her or the children? Has he killed or attacked pets? Is he extremely jealous or possessive? Does he have access to weapons? Is he depressed, despondent, or paranoid? Does he stalk her? Are his actions escalating? What is his criminal record? Does he chronically abuse substances? Has he been violent toward the children or toward nonfamily members? Does he use pornography? (These additional indicators of danger are based on Weisz et. al, 2000; Campbell et al., 1998; Holtzworth-Munroe & Stuart, 1994; Koss et al., 1994; Demare, Briere, & Lips, 1988.)

2. *History of physical abuse toward the children.* As discussed above, abusers are more likely than nonabusers to physically abuse children, and this risk may increase postseparation. It is therefore important to evaluate a man's historical approach to discipline, including his reactions when angry at the children. Additional relevant questions include: Does he spank the children? Has he ever left marks? Does he ever grab the children roughly? Has he been involved in fights (including any that appeared mutual) with his older children? Does he minimize or justify physically abusive behaviors he has used in the past?

3. *History of sexual abuse or boundary violations toward the children.* As discussed above, there is a substantial overlap between domestic violence and incest perpetration. Evidence of sexual abuse should therefore be treated with particular care in domestic violence cases. Subtler boundary violations can also be psychologically destructive and can create a context for future sexual abuse or be signs of current undisclosed sexual abuse (Salter, 1995). Questions to explore include: Does the abuser respect his children's right to privacy and maintain proper privacy himself? Does he expose the children to pornography? Does he pressure the children for unwanted physical affection or engage them in inappropriate sexual conversation? Does he make inappropriate comments about the children's bodies or physical development? Are there indications of secret keeping?

4. *Level of psychological cruelty to the mother or the children.* Our clinical experience indicates that an abuser's history of mental cruelty toward the mother or the children is an important indicator of how his conscience operates and in turn how safe children will be in his care. Re-

search indicates that the degree of emotional abuse in the home is an important determinant of the severity of difficulties developed by children exposed to domestic violence (Hughes, Graham-Bermann, & Gruger, 2001). A history of cruelty is overlooked in many evaluations, despite the fact that a majority of abused women report that the perpetrator's psychological abuse is even more destructive than his physical violence (Follingstad et al., 1990). Questions to explore include: What have been his most emotionally hurtful acts toward the mother? What behaviors of his have caused the greatest distress to the children? Has he ever deliberately harmed the children emotionally?

5. *Level of coercive or manipulative control exercised during the relationship.* We find that the more severely controlling our clients are toward their partners, the more likely they are to draw the children in as weapons of the abuse and the more likely they are to be authoritarian fathers. Additionally, a dictatorial level of control over children is associated with increased risk of both physical abuse (review in Milner & Chilamkurti, 1991) and sexual abuse (Leberg, 1997; Salter, 1995). Relevant questions include: Has he interfered with her social or professional contacts? Is he economically coercive? Does he dictate major decisions, showing contempt or disregard for her opinions? Does he monitor her movements? Is he dictatorial or minutely controlling toward the children? Manipulation as a form of control can be examined through such questions as: Does he play the role of victim in the relationship? Does he abruptly switch to kind and loving behavior when he wishes to achieve certain goals? Has he sown divisions within the family? Is there evidence that he is frequently dishonest? Is he described by his partner, children, or other witnesses as "crazy-making"? In cases where the abuser has a severe or chronic problem with lying, children's safety can be compromised by his ability to cover up the realities of his parenting behavior. Such a perpetrator may also lie directly to the children about their mother, which can create confusion for them or foster tensions in their relationships with their mother. Evaluators should thus always examine evidence of an abuser's credibility.

6. *Level of entitlement and self-centeredness.* "Entitlement" refers to an abuser's perception of himself as deserving of special rights and privileges within the family (Silverman & Williamson, 1997; Pence & Paymar, 1993; Edleson & Tolman, 1992). It can be manifested through a selfish focus on his own needs, the enforcement of double standards, a view of family members as personal possessions, or self-centered grandiosity regarding his qualities as a partner or as a parent that contrasts with evidence of his abusiveness. Self-centeredness increases the chance of violent reoffending in abusers (Saunders, 1995; Tolman & Bennett, 1990). Furthermore, our clinical experience is that the perpetra-

tor who is particularly high in entitlement tends to chronically exercise poor parenting judgment and to expect children to take care of his needs. These observations are also consistent with indications that propensity to perpetrate incest is linked to self-centeredness (Leberg, 1997; Bresee, Stearns, Bess, & Packer, 1986), a view of the children as owned objects (Salter, 1995), and attitudes of paternal entitlement (Hanson, Gizzarelli, & Scott, 1994). Relevant questions in this area include: Is the abuser frequently and unreasonably demanding, becoming enraged or retaliatory when he is not catered to? Does he define the victim's attempts to defend herself as abuse of him? Does he have double standards regarding his conduct and that of other family members? Does he appear to view the children as owned objects?

7. *History of using the children as weapons, and of undermining the mother's parenting.* We have observed that abusers who have histories of chronically using children as weapons against their mother, or of deliberately undermining her parenting, usually continue or intensify those behaviors after the relationship breaks up; postseparation improvement in this regard is rare. Questions to pursue include: Has the perpetrator mistreated the children out of anger at the mother? Has he taught them negative beliefs about her? Has he ever prevented her from caring for a child? Has he ever threatened to harm, kidnap, or take custody of the children? Has he used the children to frighten her, such as by driving recklessly with them in the car? Has he threatened to quit his job in order to avoid paying child support? Does he involve the children in activities that he knows the mother does not permit, or undermine her authority in other ways?

8. *History of placing children at physical or emotional risk while abusing their mother.* We find that an abuser's behaviors that have the effect of harming or endangering children during partner abuse, even if the children were not intended targets, can demonstrate that his determination to abuse the mother sometimes overrides his use of safe parenting judgment. This type of reckless insistence on gaining retribution against the mother increases postseparation in some cases, with attendant augmented risk to children. Abusers who are violent in the presence of children have also been found to be more physically dangerous (Thompson, Saltzman, & Johnson, 2001). Relevant questions include: Has the abuser been violent or mentally cruel during any of the mother's pregnancies? Has he been violent in the presence of the children, assaulted her while a child was in her arms, or pushed a child out of his way to get at her? Has he ever thrown objects in a way that has risked hitting the children? Has he verbally abused or humiliated the mother in the children's presence? Has he neglected the children when angry at her?

9. *History of neglectful or severely underinvolved parenting.* An

abuser's history of lack of proper attention to his children's needs is particularly relevant in the postseparation context. Additionally, studies indicate that a father's very low involvement in parenting during a child's early years increases his statistical risk of perpetrating incest (Milner, 1998). Relevant questions include: Does the perpetrator have a history of disappearing for hours, days, or weeks at a time? Has he ever refused to attend to children's medical needs? Has his lack of attentiveness ever put the children in danger? Has he shown an abrupt interest in the children, perhaps including seeking custody, in response to the dissolution of the parental relationship? The abuser's own knowledge and compassion regarding children should be tested with such questions as: Can you tell me the names of your children's current and past teachers? Could you describe each child's infancy? What are each child's particular interests, likes, and dislikes? What struggles is each child currently encountering? What kind of involvement do you maintain with any children you have from past relationships?

10. *Refusal to accept the end of the relationship or to accept the mother's decision to begin a new relationship.* An abuser's refusal to accept his partner's decision to leave him, which often is accompanied by severe jealousy and possessiveness, is linked to increased danger (Weisz et al., 2000), including danger of homicide (Websdale, 1999), putting children at increased risk. We observe clinically that those abusers who have high levels of these tendencies often also show increased use of children as tools of abuse or control postseparation. Finally, even those perpetrators who welcome the end of a relationship should be evaluated for their level of desire to punish the mother for perceived transgressions from the past or to establish paternal dominion over the children. Relevant questions include: Is the abuser depressed or panicked about the breakup, or insisting that the relationship is not over? Is he stalking her? Did he abruptly demand custody or expanded visitation upon learning that the mother had decided definitively not to go back to him, or when she began a new romantic involvement? Has he ever threatened or assaulted a new partner of hers, or warned her not to let any man other than him be around the children? Has he attempted to frighten the children about the mother's new partner, or to induce guilt in them for developing an attachment to him?

11. *Level of risk for abduction of the children.* The elevated risk of abduction by an abuser, particularly in cases where he has made related threats, was described earlier. Even in the absence of threats, evaluators should investigate indications such as abrupt passport renewals or efforts to get the children's passports away from the mother, surprise appearances at the children's schools, job seeking in other states or countries, or unexplained travel plans.

12. *Substance abuse history.* Perpetrators who abuse substances are at an increased risk to physically abuse children (Suh & Abel, 1990), to reoffend violently against the mother (Gondolf, 1998; Woffordt et al., 1994), and to commit homicide (Websdale, 1999; Campbell, 1995). Substance abuse is also linked to increased risk of perpetrating sexual abuse (Becker & Quinsey, 1993). Even in cases where the abuser states he has overcome substance abuse, evaluators need to carefully examine the length and depth of the abuser's recovery, including his level of insight regarding the addiction, and should make sure that proper ongoing treatment and self-help are in place. Additionally, any tendency on the abuser's part to blame his violence on the addiction should be treated as a sign of risk for the future, even if he is in recovery.

13. *Mental health history.* Although mental illness is found in only a minority of abusers (Gondolf, 1999), even among those who kill (Websdale, 1999), such problems when present can increase the danger of a perpetrator (Websdale, 1999; Campbell et al., 1998) and his resistance to change (Edleson & Tolman, 1992). Certain diagnoses such as antisocial personality disorder, obsessive–compulsive disorder, major depression, and borderline personality disorder have been important contributors to danger in some of our cases. A mentally ill abuser needs proper separate interventions for his abusiveness and for his psychological difficulties. The absence of mental illness or personality disorder, however, reveals little about an abuser's likelihood to be a safe or responsible parent. Psychological tests and evaluations do not predict parenting capacity well, even in the absence of domestic violence (Brodzinsky, 1994). Furthermore, mental health testing cannot distinguish an abuser from a nonabuser (O'Leary, 1993), assess the danger of abusers (APA Presidential Task Force on Violence and the Family, 1996), or measure propensity to perpetrate incest (Milner, 1998; Myers, 1997). Psychological evaluation with abusers is therefore useful only for ruling out psychiatric concerns.

For case examples illustrating the above 13 areas to be explored, see Bancroft and Silverman (2002).

In collecting and evaluating evidence regarding these indicators of risk, evaluators should pay particularly close attention to the knowledge and perceptions of the abused mother. We find that failure to do so is one of the most common weaknesses in risk assessments in domestic violence cases, particularly in custody and visitation evaluations. In cases where the perpetrator is still living in the home, the evaluator needs to develop a cooperative relationship with the abused mother to the greatest extent possible, understanding that proper compassion, support, and services for her are in most cases the key to building safety for her children (Magen, 1999; Whitney & Davis, 1999). Additionally, we wish to caution evaluators against making assumptions about level of risk to children based on the economic class, race, or level of education of the abuser. We repeatedly encounter cases where courts and child protective services have underestimated the physical, sexual, or psychological danger to children from abusers who are well educated and professionally successful. We also observe cases where risk from minority abusers has been exaggerated, particularly if they are also low-income.

Evaluators need to be prepared to conceptualize each abuser's parenting as falling on a continuum, and use multiple sources of information to evaluate where on that continuum he appears to fall. It can be helpful to think of three separate dimensions of risk, as a perpetrator may be found to have one level of physical danger to his children, another level of sexual danger, and yet another of psychological danger. We discourage the use of models that attempt to assess risk to children by placing abusers in distinct types, as such models lack both clinical and research bases at this time (see analysis of Johnston & Campbell, 1993, in Bancroft & Silverman, 2002).

Bancroft and Silverman (2002) offer detailed guidelines regarding custody and visitation planning in domestic violence cases. As discussed, the physical and emotional safety of both mothers and children needs to be paramount in such plans, along with the need to create a healing context that can support children's resilience.

ASSESSING CHANGE IN ABUSERS

Evaluators sometimes need to determine the validity of an abuser's claim that he has overcome his problem with abusiveness. Such a determination requires a clear understanding of the nature of the problem. The roots of domestic violence are a definable set of attitudes, beliefs, and behavioral patterns. These characteristics include, among others, the man's belief in his right to use violence against a partner to impose his will (Silverman & Williamson, 1997), his sense of entitlement within the family (Edleson & Tolman, 1992), his patterns of controlling and manipulative behaviors (Lloyd & Emery, 2000), disrespect for his partner and lack of empathy for her feelings (Russell & Frohberg, 1995; Pence & Paymar, 1993), and his externalizing of responsibility for his actions (Dutton, 1995). We have been involved in a number of cases where an evaluator has expressed his or her belief that an abuser has changed, despite multiple indications of lack of progress in overcoming any of the qualities that foster domestic violence. Assessment of change in an abuser therefore should draw on multiple sources of information (not

just the abuser's self-report), and include attention to the following issues, at a minimum.

Has He Made Full Disclosure of His History of Physical and Psychological Abuse?

A perpetrator must overcome denial and minimization to meaningfully
confront his abusive behavior (Adams, Bancroft, German, & Sousa,
1992; see Leberg, 1997, on the similar dynamic in treating child sexual
abusers). It is common for abusers to claim to have changed while simultaneously denying most of the history of violence, and a skeptical view
should be taken of such assertions.

Has He Recognized That Abusive Behavior Is Unacceptable?

We find that some perpetrators who claim to have changed continue to
justify their past violent or abusive behavior, usually through blaming
the victim, thereby leaving an opening for using such justifications for
future abuse. One indication of an abuser who may be making serious
progress is his unqualified statements that his behavior was wrong.

Has He Recognized That Abusive Behavior Is a Choice?

Some abusers may acknowledge that abuse is wrong but make the ex-
cuse that they lost control, were intoxicated, or were in emotional distress. Acceptance of full responsibility is indispensable for change (Adams et al., 1992), and needs to include recognition that abuse is
intentional and instrumental (Pence & Paymar, 1993).

Does He Show Empathy for the Effects of His Actions on His Partner and Children?

As evidence of change, an abuser should be able to identify in detail the
destructive impact his abuse has had (Pence & Paymar, 1993), and demonstrate that he feels empathy for his victims (Mathews, 1995; Edleson
& Tolman, 1992), without shifting attention back to his own emotional
injuries, grievances, or excuses.

Can He Identify His Pattern of Controlling Behaviors and Entitled Attitudes?

In order to change, an abuser has to see that his violence grows out of a
surrounding context of abusive behaviors and attitudes (Pence & Pay-

mar, 1993). He must be able to name the specific forms of abuse he has relied on (Edleson & Tolman, 1992) and the entitled beliefs that have driven those behaviors (Bancroft, 2002).

Has He Replaced Abuse with Respectful Behaviors and Attitudes?

A changing abuser responds respectfully to his (ex-)partner's grievances, meets his responsibilities, and stops focusing exclusively on his own needs. He develops nonabusive attitudes, including accepting his (ex-)partner's right to be angry (Bancroft, 2002) and reevaluating his distortedly negative view of her as a person. Attitudinal changes are important predictors of behavioral improvement in abusers (Gondolf, 2000).

Is He Willing to Make Amends in a Meaningful Way?

We have observed that perpetrators who are making genuine change develop a sense of long-term indebtedness toward their victims. This sense includes feeling responsible to lay their own grievances aside because of the extent of injury that the abuse has caused.

Does He Accept the Consequences of His Actions?

Our clients who make substantial progress come to recognize that abusive behavior rightly carries consequences with it, which may include the woman's decision to end the relationship or the placement of restrictions on the abuser's access to his children. On the other hand, continued anger or externalizing of responsibility regarding such consequences tends to portend a return to abusive behavior.

(For a more detailed guide to assessing change in abusers, see Bancroft and Silverman, 2002).

SUMMARY AND CONCLUSIONS

Children exposed to domestic violence can benefit tremendously when professionals have knowledge of the range of risks that abusers present to children and when a systematic risk assessment tool is applied by child protective services and family courts. It is our hope that the model we are proposing here can serve as a launching point for the development of increasingly refined and sophisticated approaches to protecting children exposed to men who abuse and to fostering their healing.

REFERENCES

Adams, D. (1991). *Empathy and entitlement: A comparison of battering and nonbattering husbands.* Unpublished doctoral dissertation, Northeastern University, Boston, MA. (Available from Emerge, 2380 Massachusetts Ave., Cambridge, MA, 02140)

Adams, D., Bancroft, L., German, T., & Sousa, C. (1992). *First-stage groups for men who batter.* Cambridge, MA: Emerge.

American Psychological Association Presidential Task Force on Violence and the Family. (1996). *Violence and the family.* Washington, DC: American Psychological Association.

Bancroft, L. (2002). *Why does he do that: Inside the minds of angry and controlling men.* New York: Putnam.

Bancroft, L., & Silverman, J. (2002). *The batterer as parent: Addressing the impact of domestic violence on family dynamics.* Thousand Oaks, CA: Sage.

Becker, J., & Quinsey, V. (1993). Assessing suspected child molesters. *Child Abuse and Neglect, 17,* 169–174.

Bow, J. N., & Quinnell, F. A. (2001). Psychologists' current practices and procedures in child custody evaluations: Five years after the American Psychological Association guidelines. *Professional Psychology: Research and Practice, 32*(3), 261–268.

Bowker, L., Arbitell, M., & McFerron, R. (1988). On the relationship between wife beating and child abuse. In K. Yllo & M. Bograd (Eds.), *Feminist perspectives on wife abuse* (pp. 159–174). Newbury Park, CA: Sage.

Bresee, P., Stearns, G., Bess, B., & Packer, L. (1986). Allegations of child sexual abuse in child custody disputes: A therapeutic assessment model. *American Journal of Orthopsychiatry, 56*(4), 560–569.

Brodzinsky, D. (1994). On the use and misuse of psychological testing in child custody evaluations. *Professional Psychology: Research and Practice, 24*(2), 213–219.

Campbell, J. (1995). Prediction of homicide of and by battered women. In J. Campbell (Ed.), *Assessing dangerousness.* Thousand Oaks, CA: Sage.

Campbell, J., Soeken, K., McFarlane, J., & Parker, B. (1998). Risk factors for femicide among pregnant and non-pregnant women. In J. Campbell (Ed.), *Empowering survivors of abuse: Health care for battered women and their children* (pp. 90–97). Thousand Oaks, CA: Sage.

Demare, D., Briere, J., & Lips, H. (1988). Violent pornography and self-reported likelihood of sexual aggression. *Journal of Research in Personality, 22,* 140–153.

Doyne, S., Bowermaster, J., Meloy, R., Dutton, D., Jaffe, P., Temko, S., & Mones, P. (1999). Custody disputes involving domestic violence: Making children's needs a priority. *Juvenile and Family Court Journal, 50*(2), 1–12.

Dutton, D. (1995). *The domestic assault of women: Psychological and criminal justice perspectives.* Vancouver, BC: University of British Columbia Press.

Edleson, J., & Tolman, R. (1992). *Intervention for men who batter: An ecological approach.* Newbury Park, CA: Sage.

Erickson, J., & Henderson, A. (1998). Diverging realities: Abused women and their children. In J. Campbell (Ed.), *Empowering survivors of abuse: Health care for battered women and their children* (pp. 138–155). Thousand Oaks, CA: Sage.

Finkelhor, D., Hotaling, G., & Sedlak, A. (1990). *Missing, abducted, runaway, and thrownaway children in America: First report: Numbers and characteristics, national incidence studies.* Washington, DC: U.S. Dept. of Justice.

Fleury, R., Sullivan, C., & Bybee, D. (2000). When ending the relationship does not end violence: Women's experiences of violence by former partners. *Violence Against Women, 6*(12), 1363–1383.

Follingstad, D., Rutledge, L., Berg, B., Hause, E., & Polek, D. (1990). The role of emotional abuse in physically abusive relationships. *Journal of Family Violence, 5(2),* 107–120.

Gondolf, E. (1998). Do batterer programs work? A 15 month follow-up of multi-site evaluation. *Domestic Violence Report, 3*(5), 65–66, 78–79.

Gondolf, E. (1999). MCMI-III results for batterer program participants in four cities: Less "pathological" than expected. *Journal of Family Violence, 14*(1), 1–17.

Gondolf, E. (2000). How batterer program participants avoid reassault. *Violence Against Women, 6*(11), 1204–1222.

Graham-Bermann, S. (1998). The impact of woman abuse on children's social development: Research and theoretical perspectives. In G. Holden, R. Geffner, & E. Jouriles (Eds.), *Children exposed to marital violence: Theory, research, and applied issues* (pp. 21–54). Washington, DC: American Psychological Association.

Greif, G., & Hegar, R. (1993). *When parents kidnap.* New York: Free Press.

Hanson, R. K., Gizzarelli, R., & Scott, H. (1994). The attitudes of incest offenders: Sexual entitlement and acceptance of sex with children. *Criminal Justice and Behavior, 21*(2), 187–202.

Heller, S., Larrieu, J., D'Imperio, R., & Boris, N. (1998). Research on resilience to child maltreatment: Empirical considerations. *Child Abuse and Neglect, 23*(4), 321–338.

Holden, G., & Ritchie, K. (1991). Linking extreme marital discord, child rearing, and child behavior problems: Evidence from battered women. *Child Development, 62,* 311–327.

Holtzworth-Munroe, A., & Stuart, G. (1994). Typologies of male batterers: Three subtypes and the differences among them. *Psychological Bulletin, 116*(3), 476–497.

Hughes, H., Graham-Bermann, S., & Gruger, G. (2001). Resilience in children exposed to domestic violence. In S. Graham-Bermann & J. Edleson (Eds.), *Domestic violence in the lives of children: The future of research, intervention, and social policy* (pp. 67–90). Washington, DC: American Psychological Association.

Hughes, H., & Marshall, M. (1995). Advocacy for children of battered women. In E. Peled, P. Jaffe, & J. Edleson (Eds.), *Ending the cycle of violence: Community responses to children of battered women* (pp. 121–144). Thousand Oaks, CA: Sage.

Hurley, D. J., & Jaffe, P. (1990). Children's observations of violence: II. Clinical implications for children's mental health professionals. *Canadian Journal of Psychiatry, 35*(6), 471–476.

Jacobson, N., & Gottman, J. (1998). *When men batter women: New insights into ending abusive relationships.* New York: Simon & Schuster.

Jaffe, P., & Geffner, R. (1998). Child custody disputes and domestic violence: Critical issues for mental health, social service, and legal professionals. In G. Holden, R. Geffner, & E. Jouriles (Eds.), *Children exposed to marital violence: Theory, research, and applied issues* (pp. 371–408). Washington, DC: American Psychological Association.

Jaffe, P., Wolfe, D. A., & Wilson, S. (1990). *Children of battered women.* Thousand Oaks, CA: Sage.

Johnston, J., & Campbell, L. (1993). A clinical typology of interparental violence in disputed-custody divorces. *American Journal of Orthopsychiatry, 63*(2), 190–199.

Kolbo, J., Blakely, E., & Engleman, D. (1996). Children who witness domestic violence: A review of empirical literature. *Journal of Interpersonal Violence, 11*(2), 281–293.

Koss, M., Goodman, L., Browne, A., Fitzgerald, L., Keita, G. P., & Russo, N. F. (1994). *No safe haven: Male violence against women at home, at work, and in the community.* Washington, DC: American Psychological Association.

Langford, L., Isaac, N. E., & Kabat, S. (1999). *Homicides related to intimate partner violence in Massachusetts, 1991–1995.* Boston: Peace at Home.

Leberg, E. (1997). *Understanding child molesters: Taking charge.* Thousand Oaks, CA: Sage.

Lloyd, S., & Emery, B. (2000). *The dark side of courtship: Physical and sexual aggression.* Thousand Oaks, CA: Sage.

Magen, R. (1999). In the best interests of battered women: Reconceptualizing allegations of failure to protect. *Child Maltreatment, 4*(2), 127–135.

Mahoney, P., & Williams, L. (1998). Sexual assault in marriage: Prevalence, consequences, and treatment of wife rape. In J. Jasinksi & L. Williams (Eds.), *Partner violence: A comprehensive review of 20 years of research* (pp. 113–157). Thousand Oaks, CA: Sage.

Margolin, G., John, R., Ghosh, C., & Gordis, E. (1996). Family interaction process: An essential tool for exploring abusive relationships. In D. Cahn & S. Lloyd (Eds.), *Family violence from a communication perspective* (pp. 37–58). Thousand Oaks, CA: Sage.

Mathews, D. (1995). Parenting groups for men who batter. In E. Peled, P. Jaffe, & J. Edleson (Eds.), *Ending the cycle of violence: Community responses to children of battered women* (pp. 106–120). Thousand Oaks, CA: Sage.

McCloskey, L. A., Figueredo, A. J., & Koss, M. (1995). The effect of systemic family violence on children's mental health. *Child Development, 66,* 1239–1261.

McGee, C. (2000). *Childhood experiences of domestic violence.* Philadelphia: Jessica Kingsley.

McMahon, M., & Pence, E. (1995). Doing more harm than good?: Some cautions on visitation centers. In E. Peled, P. Jaffe, & J. Edleson (Eds.), *Ending the cycle of violence: Community responses to children of battered women* (pp. 186–206). Thousand Oaks, CA: Sage.

Milner, J. (1998). Individual and family characteristics associated with intrafamilial child physical and sexual abuse. In P. Trickett & C. Schellenbach (Eds.), *Violence against children in the family and community* (pp. 141–170). Washington, DC: American Psychological Association.

Milner, J., & Chilamkurti, C. (1991). Physical child abuse perpetrator characteristics: A review of the literature. *Journal of Interpersonal Violence, 6*(3), 345–366.

Myers, J. (1997). *Evidence in child abuse and neglect cases* (3rd ed., 2 vols.). New York: Wiley.

O'Leary, D. (1993). Through a psychological lens: Personality traits, personality disorders, and levels of violence. In R. Gelles & D. Loseke (Eds.), *Current controversies on family violence* (pp. 7–30). Newbury Park, CA: Sage.

Paveza, G. (1988). Risk factors in father–daughter child sexual abuse. *Journal of Interpersonal Violence, 3*(3), 290–306.

Peled, E. (1998). The experience of living with violence for preadolescent children of battered women. *Youth and Society, 29*(4), 395–430.

Peled, E. (2000). The parenting of men who abuse women: Issues and dilemmas. *British Journal of Social Work, 30,* 25–36.

Pence, E., & Paymar, M. (1993). *Education groups for men who batter: The Duluth model.* New York: Springer.

Radford, L., & Hester, M. (2001). Overcoming mother blaming: Future directions for research on mothering and domestic violence. In S. Graham-Bermann & J. Edleson (Eds.), *Domestic violence in the lives of children: The future of research, intervention, and social policy* (pp. 135–155). Washington, DC: American Psychological Association.

Russell, M. N., & Frohberg, J. (1995). *Confronting abusive beliefs: Group treatment for abusive men.* Thousand Oaks, CA: Sage.

Salter, A. (1995). *Transforming trauma: A guide to understanding and treating adult survivors of child sexual abuse.* Newbury Park, CA: Sage.

Saunders, D. (1995). Prediction of wife assault. In J. Campbell (Ed.), *Assessing dangerousness* (pp. 68–95). Thousand Oaks, CA: Sage.

Silverman, J., & Williamson, G. (1997). Social ecology and entitlements involved in battering by heterosexual college males: Contributions of family and peers. *Violence and Victims, 12*(2), 147–164.

Sirles, E., & Franke, P. (1989). Factors influencing mothers' reactions to intrafamily sexual abuse. *Child Abuse and Neglect, 13,* 131–139.

Straus, M. (1990). Ordinary violence, child abuse, and wife-beating: What do they have in common? In M. Straus & R. Gelles (Eds.), *Physical violence in American families* (pp. 403–424). New Brunswick, NJ: Transition.

Suh, E., & Abel, E. M. (1990). The impact of spousal violence on the children of the abused. *Journal of Independent Social Work, 4*(4), 27–34.

Thompson, M., Saltzman, L., & Johnson, H. (2001). Risk factors for physical injury among women assaulted by current or former spouses. *Violence Against Women, 7*(8), 886–899.

Tjaden, P., & Thoennes, N. (2000). *Extent, nature, and consequences of intimate partner violence: Findings from the National Violence Against Women Survey.* (Report No. NCJ-181867). Washington, DC: National Institute of Justice/Centers for Disease Control and Prevention.

Tolman, R., & Bennett, L. (1990). A review of quantitative research on men who batter. *Journal of Interpersonal Violence, 5*(1), 87–118.

van der Kolk, B., & McFarlane, A. (1996). The black hole of trauma. In B. van der Kolk, A. McFarlane, & L. Weisaeth (Eds.), *Traumatic stress: The effects of overwhelming experience on mind, body, and society* (pp. 3–23). New York: Guilford Press.

Websdale, N. (1999). *Understanding domestic homicide.* Boston: Northeastern University Press.

Weisz, A., Tolman, R., & Saunders, D. (2000). Assessing the risk of severe domestic violence: The importance of survivors' predictions. *Journal of Interpersonal Violence, 15*(1), 75–90.

Whitney, P., & Davis, L. (1999). Child abuse and domestic violence in Massachusetts: Can practice be integrated in a public child welfare setting? *Child Maltreatment, 4*(2), 158–166.

Williams, O., Boggess, J., & Carter, J. (2001). Fatherhood and domestic violence: Exploring the role of men who batter in the lives of their children. In S. Graham-Bermann & J. Edleson (Eds.), *Domestic violence in the lives of children: The future of research, intervention, and social policy* (pp. 157–187). Washington, DC: American Psychological Association.

Woffordt, S., Mihalic, D. E., & Menard, S. (1994). Continuities in family violence. *Journal of Family Violence, 9*(3), 195–225.

Wolak, J., & Finkelhor, D. (1998). Children exposed to partner violence. In J. Jasinksi & L. Williams (Eds.), *Partner violence: A comprehensive review of 20 years of research* (pp. 73–111). Thousand Oaks, CA: Sage.

8

Fatherhood and Domestic Violence

Exploring the Role of Abusive Men in the Lives of Their Children

OLIVER J. WILLIAMS, JACQUELYN BOGGESS, and JANET CARTER

In cases where men and women are in dispute about their relationships, additional complications develop when children are added to the mix. What is in the best interest of children when parents break up? What roles should parents and, specifically, fathers play in the lives of their children in the context of a marital dispute: breadwinner, adult male role model, and/or coequal parent? The answers to such questions are complex and cause debate from case to case. These questions become even more complicated when the father in question has been abusive to the mother of his children. Advocates in the field of domestic violence are concerned about the continuous pattern of abusive behavior by men who abuse. These men abuse women and expose children to physical and emotional abuse during the course of an intimate relationship, as well as in its aftermath (Saunders, 1994; Sheeran & Hampton, 1999; Doyne et al., 1999).

In contrast, there are also advocates who are concerned about the rights of fathers. These advocates primarily want to provide emotional support to fathers and assist them in taking responsibility for their off-spring. They encourage men to spend time with their children and address their financial and emotional needs. Many fathers face challenges in raising their children or remove themselves from the lives of their children during relationship conflicts and divorce. This disconnection between fathers and children has been referred to as an epidemic (Doherty, Kouneski, & Erickson, 1996). Advocates in this field and supporters of father involvement say that contemporary attitudes and laws involving fathers discriminate against their access to their children and capacity to parent (Doherty et al., 1996). Responsible fatherhood groups believe that today's society deemphasizes the importance of fatherhood and marriage, and that a disregard for morals has contributed to the crisis faced by children and families.

The primary goal of this chapter is to increase the reader's understanding of the concerns and challenges of the two fields. A second goal is to point out the research questions that must be addressed to be responsive to the issues faced by abused women and children exposed to violence by men who abuse who are also fathers.

FATHERHOOD: AN EMERGING MOVEMENT OF IMPORTANCE

Generally speaking, fatherhood as an emerging movement is unknown to many researchers, practitioners, and advocates in domestic violence, with the exception of perhaps fathers' rights advocates and groups. In recent years, the issue of fatherhood has received increasing attention in the nation's thinking. Many fatherhood advocates say there is a crisis in America due to the economic, physical, and emotional disconnection between fathers and their children (Blankenhorn, 1995; Popenow, 1996; Whitehead, 1993). In 1994, Vice President Al Gore held a national summit in Nashville, Tennessee, on the role of fathers in the lives of their children. Groups, organizations, members of the academic community, governmental agencies, and legislators have organized to address "responsible fatherhood" and the concerns of nonresident parents.

More children than ever before are living in a home where their father is not in residence. The reason for this trend includes the high rate of divorce: 50% of all marriages in the United States end in divorce (Cherlin, 1992). Also, one-third of all births in America are to single women, and the numbers have risen steadily over the past 30–40 years (Garfinkel,

McClanahan, Meyer, & Seltzer, 1998). There is an unprecedented increase in the number of female-headed households, which has contributed to the feminization of poverty (Doherty et al., 1996). There is also a declining presence of noncustodial fathers; 90% of children in single-parent families reside with their mothers. Within 2 years following a divorce, half of the fathers lose contact with their children (Doherty et al., 1996). Very small numbers of fathers engage and remain in the lives of their children because fathers often retreat in the face of marital conflict. In addition, for those fathers who want to remain involved in the lives of their children, many report that ex-partners, laws, and policies in this country are biased against them (Doherty et al., 1996).

Fathers who do not live with their children on a full-time basis are, by definition, nonresident parents. Many fathers are also, by means of a legal custody determination, noncustodial parents. This second situation is the result of a court ruling that the child's mother (or some other person or institution) shall have custody of the child. Generally, the fatherhood movement emerged to address the needs of fathers who neither live with nor have custody of their children but who want to be involved and supportive in their children's lives. Given statistics about divorce and out-of-wedlock childbirth, and given that women typically have custody of the children, we are now faced with the question of how to support and encourage serious parenting and positive contributions from men who do not live with their children (Garfinkel et al., 1998).

THE FATHERHOOD MOVEMENT

The general term "movement" implies a cohesive effort by groups similarly constituted and a common goal. The fatherhood movement is more accurately characterized as a confluence of activity by various types of fathers' groups, men's groups, individual fathers, and other kinds of groups, organizations, and government agencies. These groups have overlapping agendas but also significantly different agendas, objectives, and methods. The call for father involvement now comes from many quarters: advocates for poor families, men's and fatherhood groups, government agencies, and individual men who feel alienated from their families. This section describes the various elements that make up the fatherhood field. Some in the field may disagree with these labels due to the fact that there are overlapping terms and shared philosophies. The intention is to provide a general overview of the major ideas that represent these elements of the fatherhood field.

Father Involvement Programs

Father involvement projects and organizations, encouraged by the federal government, are designed to help fathers find employment and reorder their lives so they will be able to meet the financial, emotional, and physical responsibilities of raising their children. Some poor fathers believe that they have been crowded out of parenting opportunities and responsibilities by the social welfare and child support systems (Johnson, Levine, & Doolittle, 1998). Families experiencing poverty and social isolation often require government assistance. Over time, and with an increased public disenchantment with welfare, there has been a move from many quarters to bring fathers back into their families so that they can provide financial assistance, thus relieving the public burden. Some agents (including some responsible fatherhood programs) would have fathers reclaim what they perceive to be a position of responsibility that has been taken over by the government through the provision of welfare.

To describe people who conduct or participate in father involvement program activities as members of a cohesive fatherhood group would be inaccurate. Rather, father involvement activities are more often centered in fatherhood programs sponsored by nonprofit community-based organizations in low-income, high-unemployment communities. Low-income fathers who participate in these programs are engaged in employment/training and peer-group support programs or, when needed, substance abuse treatment. But generally speaking, these men do not become members of a fatherhood group or organization. The fatherhood organizations provide services to help respond to the special needs of this segment of men. It should also be noted that although such programs have been targeted for men/fathers, some of them also provide similar services for female co-parents when requested.

On the one hand, father involvement advocates encourage establishing paternity and child support contributions by fathers. On the other hand, they are concerned that welfare and child support systems exacerbate barriers to father involvement among low-income families. For example, many couples who have children together do not get married but continue to live together in a family situation. They pool their emotional resources and modest financial resources to take care of their children and themselves. But the father may be legally designated as a noncustodial parent, even though he physically resides with the child and the child's mother. These fathers are not nonresident fathers, but they are, by law, noncustodial parents. Often parents faced with this reality conclude that the best thing for their children is for the mother to deny knowledge of the father's whereabouts and for the father to provide support directly to her as he is able, either in-kind or financially. Although he may actually be available, nurturing, and supportive to his child, child support and welfare systems operate to his detriment (and perhaps to the detriment of the child and mother), as if he is physically absent from his child's life.

This distinction is important in analyzing how the current child support system works. A resident noncustodial father still must pay child support (send money outside the family home) to a central child support office location. There are many valid reasons for requiring central location payment. However, if the mother in this situation is receiving welfare, the money is used to repay the government for cash assistance; if she does not receive welfare, the money eventually comes back to her. If they are both very poor and there is very little income from either of them, the precarious security of the household can be devastated by the mandatory payoff of a large portion of the total household income. For many low-income parents, whether or not the father is a resident of the household, or is on good terms with the mother, the child support enforcement system hurts rather than helps the children and their fathers (and mothers). The system sets an initial payment amount based on current circumstances, which cannot be changed quickly or efficiently when there is a change in financial circumstances for either party. The basis of father involvement programs is the belief that most fathers want to be responsible, involved, and supportive of their children to the best of their ability, but there are bureaucratic, societal, and/or family barriers that prevent involvement. Many father involvement advocates would agree with Jim Levine and Ed Pitt (1995), who outlined a strategy for community-based organizations and others interested in promoting father involvement:

- *Prevent* men from having children before they are ready for the financial and emotional responsibilities of fatherhood.
- *Prepare* men for the legal, financial, and emotional responsibilities of fatherhood.
- *Establish* paternity at childbirth, so that every father and child has, at a minimum, a legal connection.
- *Involve* men who are fathers, whether married or not, in an emotional connection to and financial support of their children.
- *Support* fathers in the variety of their roles and in their connection with their children, regardless of their legal and financial status (married, unmarried, employed, and unemployed).

In a 1995 research and evaluation project, the federal Department of Health and Human Services visited and interviewed practitioners working at five community-based organizations with fatherhood programs. In the resulting report, one common theme emerged: to be effective and responsible fathers, men needed first to develop the capacity to take care of themselves (U.S. Department of Health and Human Services, 1997). Unlike the two groups discussed below, the inclination of those who support father involvement is to respect a mother's life choices and to acknowledge the impact of a father's situation and his actions on both mother and child. Some fatherhood involvement programs are reluctant to address domestic violence directly in their programming for fear it will reduce the number of men seeking help from such programs. In contrast, other programs have developed relationships with battered women's programs and batterers treatment programs to attend to issues associated with domestic violence that exist among those people whom they serve.

Responsible Fatherhood Groups

The word "responsible" signals the basic moral tenor of these organizations. The call is for men to assume their moral responsibility as fathers and husbands. This group represents fathers from any socioeconomic level. Two of the most visible responsible fatherhood organizations are the Institute for American Values and the National Fatherhood Initiative. According to David Blankenhorn, director of the Institute for American Values and author of *Fatherless America*, "After divorce, when the biological father no longer lives in the house and the mother has custody (whether or not there is access or liberal visitation), the children are left 'fatherless' " (Blankenhorn, 1995, p. 36). Responsible fatherhood organizations contend that the absence of fathers in families and the inadequacy of the parenting in "female-headed" households have led to dysfunctional families and a dysfunctional society. According to Travis Ballard of the National Congress for Fathers and Families, "more than any other single factor, the absence of biological fathers is the leading cause of many of our nation's problems. Crime, drug problems, teen violence, inner-city strife, and juvenile delinquency are cited among the results of fatherless homes. The compelling implication of these findings is clear: one parent is simply not enough" (Ballard, 1995).

The National Fatherhood Initiative (NFI) is a "social movement" created to "restore responsible fatherhood as a national priority" (National Fatherhood Initiative newsletter). According to NFI's analysis of sociological and demographic statistics:

- 80% of suicidal youth come from single-parent homes.
- Fatherless children are twice as likely to drop out of school.

- 70% of juveniles in state reform institutions grew up in single-parent or no-parent situations.
- 60% of America's rapists grew up in homes without fathers.
- 72% of adolescent murderers grew up without fathers.
- 80% of adolescents in psychiatric hospitals come from broken homes.

Organizations with this kind of "family values" stand (which include Promise Keepers and other religion-based organizations) use their moral and religious beliefs to support a gender-based family structure and division of labor that encourages marriage between parents.

Fathers' Rights Groups

Since the early 1960s, divorced, middle-class fathers have made definite and concerted efforts to demand "rights" for divorced fathers (Vaux, 1997). Fathers' rights organizations are composed mostly of men who are divorced from their children's mothers. Some of the common experiences and frustrations of these noncustodial fathers led them to organize to discuss common issues and challenge what they perceive as an unfair or uninformed system. They often exchange information with one another and those outside their organizations by way of the Internet. The perception of an especially angry contingent of this group is that women and the court system have conspired together against fathers. This category actually represents a collection of membership groups, since fathers' rights groups are usually founded and administered by individual leaders. Many fathers' rights groups are drawn to various high-profile divorce lawyers who write how-to books and provide seminars to explain and educate noncustodial fathers about matrimonial law (Baskerville, 1998).

Finally, there are a few larger, more influential, and well-known fathers' rights organizations toward which smaller groups gravitate. These small organizations tend to comprise the constituency and consumers of the information provided by larger, more visible organizations. Collectively, these organizations are working toward a common goal of preserving (or restoring) what they view as fathers' rights. When people outside the movement think about this issue, it is usually with the characteristics of these organizations in mind. Individually, these divorced fathers tend to have the resources and the inclination to battle in court for custody of their children. Collectively, that inclination and those resources allow them to lobby legislators and policymakers as a special interest group to level changes in matrimonial and child support laws, including a state-mandated presumption of joint physical and legal custody (or "shared parenting" as they sometimes call it).

Those men in fathers' rights groups distinguish themselves from men in father involvement programs and responsible fatherhood organizations by taking little responsibility for ending their marriages, or for conflict-ridden relationships with their wives or girlfriends, or for separation from their children. In fact, some pointedly disagree with the implication from responsible fatherhood organizations that some fathers have shirked their responsibility to their families. Steven Baskerville, a political science lecturer at Howard University, says that he appreciates the fatherhood publicity generated by David Popenow and David Blankenhorn (two leaders in the responsible fatherhood arena) but wishes that they would focus more on the fact that father absence is not always voluntary (Baskerville, 1998). Baskerville cites Sanford Braver, who shows "that it is overwhelmingly wives who initiate divorce and courts that routinely throw fathers out of their families without any grounds whatever." Baskerville says, "With the exception of convicted criminals, no group in our society has fewer rights than fathers. Not just divorced fathers, not never-married fathers: fathers."

Divorced fathers voice many reasons for feeling resentment toward their former spouses and alienation from their children. Some of the early fathers' rights organizations sprouted from grassroots efforts of one or more fathers, who believe that the family court system, the child support system, and divorce policy are unfair to men and biased in favor of women (Doyne et al., 1999). Most of these organizations believe that, in particular, the child support system is unfair to noncustodial parents.

FATHERHOOD FACTIONS AND
DOMESTIC VIOLENCE PERSPECTIVES

Generally speaking, fatherhood groups view violence between intimate partners as a result of conflict and negative interactions between men and women. To some, the natural result of such conflict is violence. There are distinctions among the groups concerning their willingness to acknowledge and respond to male violence.

Father Involvement Advocates

Most father involvement supporters strongly and sincerely denounce individual acts of violence. However, their inclination is to explain violence as a result of, and a reaction to, a man's own feeling of powerlessness and inefficacy as an individual. They tend to expend the bulk of resources and concentration on addressing a father's social and personal problems. They say that the most effective way to improve a man's family life and to stop the violence is to help him change his life and get rid of those feelings of powerlessness—get him a job and a good reputation in the community, then the violence will stop.

Responsible Fatherhood Groups

This faction of the fatherhood movement acknowledges that domestic violence happens, but it suggests that blame should be placed on society and on the move away from traditional family values. It propagandizes that men's biological makeup makes them naturally aggressive and uncivilized (Blankenhorn, 1995) and that women and children pacify and tame them. However, these groups say that when the family breaks down or when society allows men to dissociate themselves from families, and when men are no longer expected to be accountable for the welfare of a family, they revert to a more savage (violent) state.

Blankenhorn (1995) contends that there is some research that suggests there is significantly less violence between married couples as compared to unmarried couples and that marriage reduces the chance that a man will be violent. He says that "the institutional inhibitor of male violence is married fatherhood" and interprets research to provide "extensive evidence which shows that the weakening of marriage and fatherhood are the principal causes of domestic violence. The connection with mothers and children give order and meaning to men's lives."

The Children's Rights Council is an organization that "seeks means of strengthening families during marriage [and] if divorce occur[s] [they] work for custody reform . . . substituting conciliation and mediation for adversarial litigation." An article in the organization's newsletter, entitled "Locating Missing and Hidden Children," states: "Local officials are used to thinking only in terms of finding parents who owe financial child support, so some of them aren't ready yet to find children being hidden by the custodial parent" (Children's Rights Council, 1999, p. 2). The article does not acknowledge that sexual abuse or partner abuse actually occurs and that women's and children's safety is a sufficient rationale for actions associated with protection.

Some policies that support responsible fatherhood do not take domestic violence into account at all. This is especially evident in discussions about women and families who receive welfare benefits. In a written statement to the White House, Travis Ballard, president of the National Congress for Fathers and Children, makes a policy recommendation strongly supporting the cooperation requirement of the welfare law (Ballard, 1995). This requires women who are not married to the father of their children to provide the father's name and identifying information for use in paternity establishment and collection of child support. Ballard makes this recommendation without reference to domestic violence. He further suggests specifically that "prior to issuance of any government aid, the party applying for the subsidy produce an affidavit from the other parent and themselves indicating that no other child care is available from the father, other relatives, or grandparents." Finally, he suggests that "when there is a genuine need for the subsidy, applicable policies should be reformulated to ensure that the father remains in the home after the birth of children and require both parties to actively participate in their children's raising and care. This might include marriage and taxpayer savings." But, clearly, in situations in which a man has been continuously violent and dangerous to his partner and children, this kind of exchange is not advised.

Representatives of the National Fatherhood Initiative contend that initiatives promoting fatherhood and marriage are often in conflict with those that seek to support single mothers achieve self-sufficiency through work.

Even when there is some lip service paid to the issue of domestic violence, there is no real respect for the contention that public policy should be made with this important issue in mind. Proponents of this viewpoint hold that although no one wants to go back to a period in human history where women (or men) could be physically or sexually abused by their spouses, and not have any escape from that abuse, divorce should be made less easy to obtain. However, if we do make it "less easy to obtain," how can we protect women who are victims of the abuse? Members of this group continue to say that they acknowledge that there is domestic violence and that abused women should be protected. In fact, they admit that some of their policy suggestions would create an environment that would put abused women at more risk, and that those women and their children should be protected. However, they never address how to do both things at once.

Fathers' Rights Groups

These fathers tend to be angry at the child's mother and at the system. Many of these groups deny that domestic violence is prevalent enough to warrant a concerted effort to deal with it. In fact, some fathers' rights groups contend that men are the victims of domestic violence at least as often as women are (Baskerville, 1998). These groups often imply that charges of violence perpetrated by men against women are fabricated or exaggerated to intimidate men and strip them of their rights as fathers.

According to Walter G. Vaux (1997), whose article appears on the website of the National Coalition of Free Men (NCFM), "Until the current trend of sequestering fathers is reversed, the nation will be crippled with dysfunctional children, weakened households, and abused men." He also implies that we should be concerned about some innate and unavoidable violence from women. Vaux refers to Paul Herzog, who "explains, on the dangerous practices arising with a single parent, that two parents provide checks. In the father's absence, the mother loses this protection, and the mother's aggressive and libidinous inclinations center on the child." Vaux (1997) also mentions a Children's Rights Coalition survey of state child protective service agencies, which found that mothers abuse children at a rate almost double that of men. In a "guest editorial" at the same website, Hughes generally ridicules and attempts to discredit advocates for victims of domestic violence. He suggests that statistics about domestic violence in his state, New Hampshire, are exaggerated and in some cases fabricated. He accuses advocates of "shameless skewing of the numbers" in order to secure federal grant money.

THE CONCERNS OF DOMESTIC VIOLENCE ADVOCATES

Do the attitudes, beliefs, intentions, and policies promoted by fatherhood advocates erode domestic violence advocates' capacity to keep women safe? Through the information cited above, a general impression is that fatherhood advocates believe that feminist and abused women's advocates label all men as abusers. They also believe that these abused women's advocates view women as innocent despite their behaviors in relationships. A prevailing view is that many abused women falsely allege partner abuse as a way to gain advantage in a marital dispute in court and child custody cases. Although researchers indicate that abused women rarely falsely allege domestic violence (Jaffe & Geffner, 1998; Faller, Olafson, & Corwin, 1993; Geffner, 1997; Pagelow, 1997; Everson & Boot, 1989; Thoennes & Tjaden, 1990), many practitioners and advocates in fathering recite cases where men have been falsely accused. Another belief of fatherhood advocates is that domestic violence is a natural result of conflict between two individuals, and that women are equal contributors to the violence. The fact is that women are significantly less likely to be perpetrators of partner abuse than men are

(Saunders, 1988; Stets & Straus, 1990; Dobash, Dobash, Wilson, & Daly, 1992; Doyne et al., 1999). Relatively small numbers of women are the primary aggressors of physical abuse, and this fact must be placed in context and not used as a ploy to minimize and discredit the issues associated with violence against women (Jaffe & Geffner, 1998). Mutual violence occurs in domestic violence cases as well. Often in such cases abused women are protecting themselves from their abuser in self-defense. But this type of violence gets reported as mutual violence (Gelles & Straus, 1988; Doyne et al. 1999). The prevailing view among domestic violence prevention advocates is that violence is behavior that perpetrators choose as a method of resolving conflict or to control their partners (Gondolf, 1985; Williams, 1999). As a result, abused women's advocates are concerned with the continuous patterns of violent and abusive behavior of men who abuse women; some of those men are fathers.

To this point, fatherhood groups have not clearly identified nonviolent and nonabusive behavior toward a female partner as among the characteristics of positive fathering. Nor, generally speaking, do these advocates address abusive behavior among fathers who abuse either their wife or their children. This lack of attention gives the impression that regardless of the consequence to the family, a father must be present, at any cost. Abused women's advocates believe that it is equally important to expect healthy behavior from fathers, whether they are residential or not. The quality of the fathering relationship is as important as having a father present.

To promote the safety and well-being of abused women and children, fatherhood advocates must acknowledge abused women's unique experiences with men who abuse. What is the reality of abused women and children exposed to domestic violence? We will explore that question in the remainder of this chapter.

CREATING SAFE, STABLE ENVIRONMENTS FOR ABUSED WOMEN

It is important for fatherhood advocates to be aware of the issues and concerns of abused women to critically examine how to respond to the behavior of men who abuse who are also fathers. As indicated in Chapter 3, 30% of all women are victims of some form of abuse in an adult relationship during their lifetime (Jaffe & Geffner, 1998; Doyne et al., 1999). Men who abuse use a range of tactics to intimidate and harass their former partners and refuse to leave their homes. Abused women look to the community, the courts, and human service professionals for understanding, protection, and support. Too often this does not materialize.

A 38-year-old woman from the East Coast speaks of the terror she feels because her ex-husband will eventually get out of jail and locate her and their child. On several occasions he threatened to kill her and her family; given his history, this was not an idle threat. She is fearful that the court may encourage her to maintain a relationship with her ex-husband, if he chooses to reconnect with their child. Despite obtaining a protection order during her divorce, she received no protection or support through the court system associated with their domestic violence and divorce dispute. The criminal justice system convicted and incarcerated her abuser on weapons charges when the police found guns and explosives in his car. He was not incarcerated nor held accountable due to partner violence.

Similarly, a 50-year old woman from the West Coast recalls her ordeal as she left an abusive husband 25 years ago. She left in the middle of the night with her four boys, all under the age of 10. She remembers how her abuser seemed to manipulate the court system. Although she got custody of the kids, he would not cooperate or take on his financial responsibility despite having the means to do so. She recalls that she and her boys went homeless for a time because he would not pay child support. He vowed never to help her or his children unless she came back. She did not, and today she boasts about raising four boys who are all college graduates.

In these cases, the criminal justice system was not able to address the concerns and danger related to partner abuse. Few courts and related human service systems have the capacity to accurately assess how abused women are affected by domestic violence (Jaffe & Geffner, 1998; Doyne et al., 1999). Professionals, including judges, social workers, psychologists, and attorneys, do not have the training to understand and assess domestic violence. The role of the courts in cases of domestic violence will be discussed further in Chapters 11 and 12. To exacerbate the current state of affairs, there is an aggressive effort by some fathers' rights advocates to minimize the importance of domestic violence as it relates to women and children. These advocates are reported to encourage the tactic of blaming abused women for child abuse and neglect.

Through child custody cases, many abused women are also labeled with "malicious mother syndrome" or "alienated parent syndrome." These terms are used to describe women who choose not to cooperate with the father of their children. In certain cases, labeling is used as an attempt to discredit abused women and their ability to parent (Saunders, 1994; Faller & Devore, 1994; Jaffe & Geffner, 1998). Such labeling may also be a ploy to shift attention from an abusive husband's behavior (McMahon & Pence, 1993). In cases where the woman is a victim and is reluctant to cooperate with the man who has eroded her safety and stability, it is important to consider abuse as an influence on her choices, decisions, and capacity to provide security for herself and her children. The important fact is that our systems are not presently sensitive enough to evaluate the circumstances and unique concerns associated with male violence. If the goal of fathers' rights groups is the best interest of the children, addressing partner violence should be a common goal of the two fields. But even when children are not involved, women have the right to safe and secure lives.

SUMMARY AND CONCLUSIONS

Collaboration between advocates for abused women and advocates of the fathers' rights faction of the fatherhood movement is impossible. However, since many individuals, interest groups, advocates, and government agencies consider themselves discussants and stakeholders in the outcome of this public discussion of nonresident father and noncustodial father involvement, it is crucial that the voices of mothers and children and their advocates be clearly heard.

As we define and conduct this collaboration, the common goal between domestic violence prevention advocate groups and advocates for father involvement must be safe, healthy environments and positive family connections for children and their parents. In order to decide how these two advocates groups with different agendas can work together, these stakeholders must talk and exchange ideas and information at meetings, conferences, and collaborative projects. Domestic violence advocates and father involvement supporters must create an alliance through these conversations and information exchanges. This alliance can inform social welfare policy and, more importantly, can provide more comprehensive services for families in need. Our mutual task is daunting, and we will have to address the difficult issues that will frame and fuel our ongoing discussion.

We have three recommendations concerning issues to acknowledge and address:

1. If we are to encourage men to become active parents, we must acknowledge that men perpetrate domestic violence against women at higher rates and more frequently than visa versa. Moreover, and more specifically, if we are to construct a public policy agenda that will partic-

ularly support and encourage father involvement in low-income, never-married families, we must be mindful of the incidence of domestic violence among women who receive welfare. Research shows that incidence, and social service practitioners verify that the number of women on welfare who are or have been victims of domestic violence is significantly higher than for the general population.

2. We must remain collectively mindful that our honest and vigilant concern about violence is not an implication, and is not perceived to be an implication, that all men (or all poor men, or all men of color) are prone to this kind of violence. Great numbers of fathers have never committed violent or abusive acts against anyone in their families and would never consider such an offense, and some fathers who have been violent may never do it again. Still, in large part because we cannot be sure who will commit a violent act against a woman or child, we must continue to pay serious attention to the possibility of violence in the context of father involvement.

3. We must be willing to talk about the difficult issues on which each side maintains strong positions. On common ground, researchers in the fatherhood field suggest that fathering cannot be isolated from mothering and mothers' expectations. Mothers often mediate fathers' access to their children. The extent to which men are successful in negotiating this issue is often determined by the quality of their relationship with their children's mothers. Relationship problems between mothers and fathers typically have disastrous effects on father–child relationships. What is significant here is that the relationship between partners is viewed as an important component for healthy co-parenting, regardless of whether the couple is together or not.

There is good news to report: there are men and women finding a common ground. The Ford Foundation brought together different people from the field of domestic violence and fatherhood to discuss these issues. The group was called Common Ground. The Center for Fathers, Families, and Public Policy and the National Nonprofit Planning Center for Community Leadership were two fathering organizations represented, along with the Family Violence Prevention Fund and the Institute on Domestic Violence in the African American Community, among others. Joe Jones and his two programs, Center for Fathers, Families, and Workforce Development and Baltimore's Healthy Start Baltimore, developed a collaboration with the domestic violence program House of Ruth (also in Baltimore) to address the issue of male violence, particularly among fathers. The Center for Fathers, Families, and Public Policy, in Madison, Wisconsin, also focuses on this issue, and explores the concerns of mothers and fathers associated with violence and what mothers need from fathers who have been abusive but still have a relationship with the father. The Institute on Domestic Violence in the African American Community and the Family Violence Prevention Fund collaborated to explore this issue in the domestic violence community and fatherhood communities. Williams and Donnelly (1998) and Donnelly, Wilson, Medoros, and Williams (2000) both created a batterers' treatment curriculum with domestic violence and fatherhood components. These are examples that the work can be done and that such an alliance can develop without sacrificing the safety of abused women and children, while focusing on change and healthy behavioral standards for fathers who have a history of abuse.

REFERENCES

Ballard, T. (1995, November 27). *Meeting on supporting the role of fathers in families, the White House* (statement of Travis Ballard, president of the National Congress for Fathers and Children). Retrieved June 25, 1999, from *http://www.acfc.org/study/ballard.htm*.

Baskerville, S. (1998). Sins of the father [Review of the book *Divorced dads: Shattering the myth*]. *Fathering Magazine*. [On-line serial]. Retrieved May 27, 1999, from *http://fatheringmag.com/news/3786-Ddads.shtml*.

Blankenhorn, D. (1995). *Fatherless America: Confronting our most urgent social problem*. New York: Beacon Press.

Cherlin, A. (1992). *Marriage, divorce, remarriage*. Cambridge, MA: Harvard University Press.

Children's Rights Council. (1999, Winter). Locating missing and hidden children. *Speak Out for Children* [Newsletter], p. 2.

Dobash, R. E., Dobash, R. P., Wilson, M., & Daly, M. (1992). The myth of sexual symmetry in marital violence. *Social Problems, 39*, 71–75.

Doherty, W. J., Kouneski, E. F., & Erickson, M. F. (1996). Responsible fathering: An overview and conceptual framework. *Report for the Administration for Children and Families and the Office of the Assistant Secretary for Planning and Evaluation of the United States Department of Health and Human Services* (pp. 1–55). Washington, DC.

Donnelly, D., Smith, L., & Williams, O. J. (2002). Batterer's education curriculum for African American men. In E. Aldorando & F. Mederos (Eds.), *Programs for men who batter*. Kingston, NJ: Civic Research Institute.

Donnelly, D., Wilson, S., Medoros, F., & Williams, O. J. (2000). *Evolved battery treatment curriculum*. (Available from Planning Unit, Court Support Services Division, Judicial Branch, State of Connecticut, 860-563-7424).

Doyne, D. E., Browermaster, J. D., Meloy, J. R., Dutton, D., Jaffe, P., Temiko, S., & Monies, P. (1999, Spring). Custody disputes involving domestic violence: Making children's needs a priority. *Juvenile and Family Court Journal, 50*(2), 1–12.

Everson, M. D., & Boot, B. (1989). False allegations of sexual abuse by children and adolescents. *American Academy of Child and Adolescent Psychiatry, 28,* 230–268.

Faller, K. C., Olafson, E., & Corwin, D. (1993). Research on false allegations of sexual abuse in divorce. *APSAC Advisor, 6*(3), 1, 7–10.

Garfinkel, I., McLanahan, S., Meyer, D. & Seltzer, J. (1998). *Fathers under fire: The revolution in child support enforcement.* New York: Russell Sage Foundation.

Geffner, R. (1997). Family violence: Current issues, interventions and research. *Journal of Aggression, Maltreatment, and Trauma, 1,* 1–25.

Gelles, R., & Straus, M. (1988). *Intimate violence: The definitive study of the causes and consequences in the American Family* (pp. 18–20). New York: Simon & Schuster.

Gondolf, E. (1985). *Men who batter: An integrated approach for stopping wife abuse.* Holmes Beach, FL: Learning Publications.

Jaffe, P. G., & Geffner, R. (1998). Child custody disputes and domestic violence: Critical issues for mental health, social service, and legal professionals. In G. W. Holden, R. Geffner, & E. N. Jouriles (Eds.), *Children exposed to marital violence: Theory, research, and applied issues* (pp. 371–408). Washington DC: American Psychological Association.

Johnson, E., Levin, A., & Doolittle, F. C. (1998). *Father's fair share: Helping poor men manage child support and fatherhood.* New York: Russell Sage Foundation.

Levine, J. A., & Pitt, E. W. (1995). *New expectations: Community strategies for responsible fatherhood.* New York: Families and Work Institute.

McMahon, M., & Pence, E. (1993). Doing more harm than good?: Some cautions on visitation centers. In E. Peled, P. G. Jaffe, & J. L. Edleson (Eds.), *Ending the cycle of violence: Community responses to children of battered women* (pp. 186–206). Newbury Park, CA: Sage.

Pagelow, M. D. (1997). Battered women: A historical research review and some common myths. In R. Geffner, S. Sorrenson, & P. K. Lundberg-Love (Eds.), *Violence and sexual abuse at home: Current issues, interventions, and research in spousal battering and child maltreatment* (pp. 26–48). Binghamton NY: Haworth Maltreatment and Trauma Press.

Popenow, D. (1996). *Life without father.* New York: Pressler Press.

Saunders, D. G. (1988). Other truths about domestic violence: A reply to McNeely and Robinson-Simpson. *Social Work, 33,* 179–183.

Saunders, D. G. (1994). Child custody decisions in families experiencing women abuse. *Social Work, 39,* 51.

Sheeran, M., & Hampton, S. (1999). Supervised visitation in cases of domestic violence. *Juvenile and Family Court Journal, 50,* 13–26.

Stets, J., & Straus, M. (1990). Gender differences in reporting marital violence and its medical psychological consequences. In M. Straus & R. Gelles (Eds.), *Physical violence in American families: Risk factors and adaptations to violence* (pp. 151–166). New Brunswick, NJ: Transaction.

Thoennes, N., & Tjaden, P. (1990). The extent, nature, and validity of sexual

abuse allegations in custody/visitation disputes. *Child Abuse and Neglect,*
14, 151–163.

U.S. Department of Health and Human Services, Federal Interagency Forum on
Child and Family Statistics. (1997). *Nurturing fatherhood: Improving data
and research on male fertility, family formation, and fatherhood.* Available
online: *http://fatherhood.hhs.gov/CFSForum/front.htm.*

Vaux, W. G. (1997). *Are fathers really necessary?* Retrieved February 12, 2001,
from *http://www.ncfm.org.*

Whitehead, B. D. (1993). Dan Quayle was right. *The Atlantic Monthly.* [Online
serial]. Retrieved February 12, 2001, from *http://theatlantic.com/politics/
family/danquayl.htm.*

Williams, O. J. (1999). African American men who batter: Treatment considerations and community response. In R. Staples (Ed.), *The Black families:
Essays and studies* (6th ed., pp. 265–280). New York: Wadsworth.

Williams, O. J., & Donnelly, D. (1997). *Batterer's education curriculum for African American men.* (Available through Oliver Williams, School of Social
Work, College of Human Ecology, University of Minnesota, St. Paul, MN,
55108).

Part III

SYSTEM-LEVEL RESPONSES

9

The Ethnic Media Outreach Project

"Canada Is a Country for Women"

MELPA KAMATEROS

Part of the ethnocultural reality of Canada is the existence of a large number of people who speak neither English nor French, Canada's two official languages. According to the 2001 census, 18.4% of the Canadian population were born outside Canada, reflecting over 200 ethnicities (Statistics Canada, 2003a, 2003b). We must also take into account that the number of people who encounter language difficulties would be even higher if those who have a minimal knowledge of either English or French were added to these figures. The Ethnic Media Outreach Project was therefore developed to address the needs of the women and the communities where issues of linguistic and cultural access exist.

In Canada, the federal government implemented the Family Violence Initiative to reduce violence against women, children, and older adults. The Multiculturalism Program of Heritage Canada is part of this initiative, and works with nongovernmental organizations and ethnic media to deliver domestic violence prevention information specifically to ethnic and visible minority communities. In 1997, the Ethnic Media Outreach Project (EMOP) was funded through this initiative. Its main goal was to raise awareness in communities where linguistic and cultural barriers made access to information on both family violence and the existing services for victims very difficult. The EMOP was implemented by four community agencies in three parts of Canada, each responsible for coordinating the programs for different ethnocultural communities.

The main goal of the EMOP project is to increase public awareness of domestic violence and related resources in communities where there is little knowledge of either of Canada's official languages. The ethnic language media of the various communities concerned deliver the message, ensuring that both the content and the transmission of the messages on violence are linguistically and culturally attuned. The long-term goal of the program is to create social change through public awareness—to change how people think and act.

This chapter focuses on the Montreal project, coordinated by the Shield of Athena Family Services, a community-based social service agency serving families from Greek and other ethnocultural communities. To date, broadcasts have been done with 12 communities (Portuguese, Italian, Greek, Armenian, Egyptian, Lebanese, Haitian, South Asian, Iranian, Spanish, Chinese, and Russian), reaching close to half a million people.

SPECIFIC NEEDS OF IMMIGRANT
WOMEN AND CHILDREN

It is mostly immigrant women who speak neither of the official languages fluently. Should they also be victims of violence and want to access the police, a crisis line, or the shelters, they would be severely restricted by linguistic barriers (Roboubi & Bowles, 1995). Language barriers, however, are not the only problem. Cultural and religious issues, extended families, societal roles, and sexual stereotyping are other problems they may have to deal with. Importantly, they may also be faced with silence at the community level, as these issues are rarely discussed openly.

The daily existence of these women is permeated with *fear*—fear of deportation, fear of their husbands, fear of social castigation, fear of losing their children (because they do not know the laws), and fear of the system.

The element of choice is not available for women who do not speak the language of the host country. Since she cannot speak, she cannot act. On the other hand, even if she speaks the language, there are cultural and religious factors at play that may impede her access to services.

DOMESTIC VIOLENCE: AN INVISIBLE ISSUE IN MANY COMMUNITIES

According to information from the Shield of Athena Family Services Center, most of the clients who have been victims of family violence first go to their family or friends for help. Yet, abused women may be faced with silence at the community level, where domestic violence is not openly discussed and indeed may even be tolerated. This is not to suggest that there is more or less abuse in one ethnic community or another. Instead, the problem is focused on the silence that is kept and the barriers to disclosure that act to prevent women from seeking assistance. When people do not talk openly about an issue, they may not fully understand it; they are isolated, and they do not know where to turn for help. There is a vicious cycle in play regarding the issue of domestic violence and how it is viewed in ethnocultural communities. When people are not sensitized and informed, there are no common definitions of domestic violence. As a consequence, there is no framework for discussion and comparison. Such violence is therefore invisible. Whatever the cause, the consequence is that service providers may not see ethnocultural clients at their doors, leading them to presume there are no problems.

THEMES AND MESSAGES OF THE PROJECT

Therefore, even if the woman has the information, she may hesitate to ask for help, primarily because she lacks support at two levels:

1. Community and family level (i.e., her extended family, religious leaders, and her own children).
2. Service level (because of the lack of outreach in the ethnic tongue and specialized services to meet her needs).

Figure 9.1 shows the possible effects of ethnic outreach media programs.

The Ethnic Media Outreach Project was designed to address the

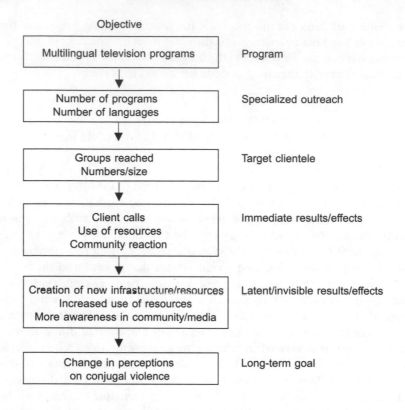

FIGURE 9.1. Possible effects of ethnic outreach media programs. Property of the Shield of Athena Family Services.

specific needs of women from ethnocultural communities. The two central themes of the campaign are to (1) address the issue of domestic violence and make it visible and (2) return responsibility for the issue to the communities. The following messages are also an integral part of the program:

- Violence is not a feminist issue, it is a human rights issue.
- Stopping the violence is everyone's concern.
- Violence has serious repercussions for children.
- Help is possible.
- Men, being part of the problem, must be part of the solution.
- There is no shame in disclosure.
- Violence is a learned behavior that is cyclical in nature.

OBTAINING COMMUNITY SUPPORT

A crucial part of the project was obtaining community support through the recruitment of professionals and political and community leaders. Their involvement and ongoing support were necessary to legitimize the issues in their communities. In addition, we entered into partnerships with other agencies whenever possible and made links with religious institutions. The ethnic media were involved in this process.

We used a number of specific strategies to obtain community support for the program, including:

- Setting up informal or formal meetings with women's groups, religious associations, private professionals, and media individuals.
- Contacting health and social service agencies to find lists of ethnocultural social workers, doctors, and psychologists.
- Contacting the police to identify officers from minority communities who would be willing to participate in the media messages.
- Contacting people associated with organizations, committees, and associations with whom we had done other projects, to obtain their insights into the communities in question.

The advantages of this process became evident as the project developed. First, by obtaining the support of all these individuals and organizations in the initial phase, we created an informal network of resource people who would, after the programs were aired, help clients or refer them to services. Second, these individuals and organizations would then have a role in the ongoing sensitization and prevention in their individual communities.

USING THE ETHNIC MEDIA

A message repeatedly heard by community agencies is that most clients who are victims of domestic violence turn to family or friends for help before going to an agency. In addition, because of linguistic issues, many communities turn to the ethnic media for programs and information in their mother tongue. Although these programs are most often used to sell products, tell people what is happening in their mother country, or import soap operas or athletic matches for their viewing audiences, we felt the ethnic media could also be used to sensitize whole communities about domestic violence.

It was a challenge to use this programming to inform people about an issue many did not want to acknowledge existed. However, we were able to use previous experiences as evidence for the positive effect the ethnic media could have in raising public awareness of domestic violence. Taking our previous experiences into consideration, we applied these principles to this larger project, and expanded the number of communities that were reached by the EMOP to 12.

INVISIBLE PROBLEM, INVISIBLE CLIENTELE

The first goal of the project was to make the problem of domestic violence visible. In Vancouver, the People's Law School produced 12 radio programs for four communities. Over the course of a year, COSTI in Toronto produced 21 radio and television programs for seven communities. In our project in Montreal, we made 25 television programs in 15 different languages during a 2-year period. Our programs deal with violence against women, child abuse, elder abuse, and children exposed to violence. For many communities, these programs were the first they had seen dealing with these topics, as these issues are rarely disclosed. In Montreal, by communicating our messages solely through the ethnic television media, the project:

- Made the issue visible, putting a face or a series of faces to it.
- Reduced or removed the shame by promoting open talk in a very public manner.
- Applied the news to everybody—no one community was singled out.
- Marketed a strategy that would go over well, in partnership and consultation with our network of community partners.

To further legitimize the project, we used excerpts of a message from the then current Secretary of State and Minister for the Status of Women, a woman belonging to a visible minority group who was herself not born in Canada. Three other Members of Parliament with ethnocultural backgrounds were also featured.

FORMAT OF THE TELEVISION PROGRAMS

All of the programs were 12–15 minutes in length. They were labor-intensive, and creating them had to take all the participants' schedules into account. Meetings, for example, took place after normal office hours or on weekends to ensure maximum participation. In addition to consultations with community partners, the time needed for scripting, translating, discussing, rehearsing, and taping the programs had to be coordinated with various participants' schedules. The programs' technical costs were high due to the nature of the issue. Translation, production, editing, and broadcast all took time and financial resources. We were unable to forge partnerships in some of the communities; therefore, other types of arrangements had to be made to validate the programs. This created problems in terms of providing services and follow-up with clients after the programs were aired.

The programs use different types of presentations: interview (Greek, Arab, Persian, Armenian communities); roundtable discussion (Portuguese, Italian); dramatizations (Chinese, Haitian); and a combination of interview and dramatization (Spanish, Russian).

Some of the programs address the issue of violence directly, while others show it indirectly. The needs and characteristics of the communities were taken into account when designing each one. Most were formally scripted and rehearsed to avoid confusion or misunderstanding on the part of the viewing audience. The program messages include:

- Violence is not acceptable.
- There is no shame in disclosure.
- Everybody is hurt by violence.
- Abuse happens everywhere.
- There are resources for men, women, and children.
- Men are part of the solution.
- The community has an obligation to inform and protect the victims of abuse.
- Laws exist to protect the victims.
- The woman is not to blame.
- Violence is the family's, the community's, and society's concern.

The cycle of violence, the forms of abuse, and the power and control model are defined in every program on conjugal violence. Initially, many members of the various communities did not even know the meaning of this term—abuse. Subsequently, the explanation of abuse using the perspective of power and control, and in simple language, was received very well by the audiences. In the programs on child and elder abuse, definitions are provided by doctors, lawyers, policemen, and social workers, to further demonstrate that such violence does not affect only women—it is not only a woman's affair—and that it is not only a "feminist" issue.

We consciously made the decision to include many men in the various segments. We hoped that by showing a variety of men discussing the issues, the viewing audience would not directly blame the male gender in general (as opposed to the abuser), and as a result reduce the defensiveness of the viewing audience. We believe that including men in different roles in the programs helped make the viewing audience more receptive to the message they were being given. In summary, we used methods and strategies that met the needs and worked for each individual ethnic community so as to assure the "made to measure" messages were as effective as possible. A whole psychology was used to determine how, what, and when messages were delivered and communicated.

COMMUNITY REACTION

Because the media messages were marketed from the perspective of the communities and were scripted and produced in the mother tongue, there was little negative community reaction. One comment that was encountered was the feeling that Canada is a country for women—that women seem to have more rights than men. Some people were surprised to find out that violence exists everywhere, including even Canada. Some asked, "Despite all these laws and resources, do Canadian men have this problem in controlling their wives, too?" Finally, we sometimes observed denial, anger, or minimization of the problem by community leaders who continued to view domestic violence as a "private family matter" or as an issue that should be relegated to "women's affairs."

There were also concerns that there were not enough services for the victims, and that the communities wanted more programs made available. A few professionals were hesitant or reluctant to speak about the issue. Some community leaders were initially surprised that domestic violence existed as a problem in their community. This was also a positive reaction, however, because it generated dialogue, thereby making the problem more visible. For this project, the strategy was important, since the program was intended for many communities in many parts of the country, and the federal government's involvement gave the initiative legitimacy and credibility.

DEVELOPING THE PUBLIC SERVICE ANNOUNCEMENT

Another phase of this project was developing a 30-second Public Service Announcement (PSA) entitled "Violence Hurts Us All," which was translated into 16 languages. It was co-produced by Rogers Cable, CFMT-TV in Toronto (a multilingual television station), and Heritage Canada, with content advice from the author. Using the same framework as the media programs, we introduced the concept of the child in the middle to emphasize the harm to children exposed to domestic violence. At the end of each of the 16 PSAs, the child questions what is happening in his or her language.

The PSA won first prize in the Television Bureau of Canada's 1999 Retail Comp Awards, from among 426 other entries. One station in Toronto, Telelatino, aired it in Spanish and Italian 300 times over 3 months. It has been aired by over 250 cable stations from coast to coast, and has been received favorably by all communities, since the message comes from the child. Most of our programs also have this PSA included as part of the message, to maximize impact. We are currently examining new strategies to rebroadcast the PSA this year, perhaps by giving it directly to the producers of ethnic programming. CH, the ethnic channel in Quebec has already included it in its programming.

LAST PHASE OF THE PROJECT

In the project's last phase, in order to better serve communities in which there is a language barrier, two videos, one on police and judicial procedure and the other on resources were produced in the following seven languages: Italian, Greek, Arab, Chinese (Mandarin), Russian, Spanish, and Portuguese (for a total of 14 videos).

The communities and languages were chosen based on the following criteria:

- Size of the community. For example, the Italian community numbers over 150,000 in Montreal.
- An interest in participating. The Russian community is small but is constantly increasing in numbers. Because of this increase, we were approached by this community to create programs since none had been made before.
- The need to serve communities that had been in Canada for a long time. For example, in certain southern European communities, such as the Portuguese or Greek community, many people still do not speak English or French, so there was a need to disseminate information in their native language. In the Chinese community, their conjugal violence program had been cut due to lack of funds, and there was a need for us to provide this program for them in their native languages (Mandarin and Cantonese).

- Many of the communities had participated in the first phase of the project. Our partners included two women's shelters, six women's centers, and one community center, as well as mainstream services, such as the Police Services of Montreal and the S.O.S. hotline. The Police Services of Montreal, in particular, were key partners in this project.

Goals of This Phase

Through the production of these two videos, we hoped to provide basic information to a number of ethnic communities on police procedure and what transpires after an initial 911 call.

In the earlier phase of this project, we met with communities on a separate basis in order to have a "made to measure" approach regarding these programs. In this phase of the project, however, since there was only one set of laws that governed police and judicial procedure and one existing network of resources that had to be explained, we just wrote one script for each video, which was then translated into the seven languages. We also met with police to provide information on the police procedure for the first video and the director of a women's shelter to provide resource information for the second video. This information was then incorporated into the scripts for each video and translated. In the second video, we also included interviews with the S.O.S. hotline and different ethnocultural community centers.

At the moment, feedback about the video program has not yet been evaluated, as we are currently perfecting a made to measure diffusion strategy in which we will gauge the program's effectiveness.

OVERVIEW OF THE EFFECTIVENESS OF THE PROGRAMS

We cannot evaluate the programs in a quantitative way, but we can judge their effectiveness in a qualitative manner. The *immediate* impact of the programs on the community was an increase in the awareness of domestic violence as an issue, as evidenced by the increased number of calls to our community partners and the media. In addition, the calls came from urban as well as rural areas, indicating the message reached a range of audiences.

We also need to consider the *latent* effects of these programs. How long will the members of the community retain the information? In this case, people call us months and even up to 1 year after the programs aired, indicating the programs may have long-lasting effects. We predict that, as a result of the response to the programs, we will start to see the creation of community organizations dealing with domestic violence where there were previously none. In addition, the communities may start to reuse the programs as educational tools. Finally, we have observed the ongoing interest of the ethnic media in terms of commenting on and producing programs about this issue. This extension of the programs and continued focus are important for prevention and sensitization of communities.

These programs may also have an *invisible* impact, including the increased use of mainstream resources (impossible for us to assess in the scope of this project). The eventual creation of infrastructures and community resources are also important aftereffects of these programs. For example, the ethnic media have become important allies with service organizations. Very often the media were bombarded with calls and requests after broadcasting the programs. Many producers became our S.O.S. line, referring clients to professionals, community organizations, and existing resources. They also began to read the news more avidly and incorporated programs on domestic violence of their own volition.

In general, the programs caused an initial chain reaction, a catalyst effect that promoted the integration of the communities in Canadian society through more knowledge of the issues, legislation, and resources.

SUMMARY AND CONCLUSIONS

Our experience with the Ethnic Media Outreach Project demonstrates that community outreach can work to raise public awareness of domestic violence among communities that differ linguistically and culturally from the dominant society. Specifically, we learned that:

- The ethnic media is the best channel for transmitting information to ethnocultural communities.
- In order to be effective, ethnic broadcasting should be continuous.
- Information on existing resources and the laws should be available in many languages.

We cannot wait for minority communities to come looking for the news. We must use their cultural language for such sensitization to be effective. As such, and within the scope of our particular project, we emphasize the need for continuing public education: knowledge is power; power is choice, and choice is action. Power is freedom from the shackles of such violence for us all—men, women, and future generations. The media, as an educational tool, has one of the greatest roles to play.

REFERENCES

Roboubi, N., & Bowles, S. (1995). *Barriers to justice: Ethnocultural minority women and domestic violence—a preliminary discussion paper.* Ottawa: Research and Statistics Division, Department of Justice Canada.

Statistics Canada (2003a, January 21). *Census of population: Immigration, birthplace and birthplace of parents, citizenship, ethnic origin, visible minorities and Aboriginal peoples. The Daily.*

Statistics Canada (2003b). *Canada's ethnocultural portrait: The changing mosaic.* Ottawa: Statistics Canada (*www.statcan.ca*).

10

Police in the Lives of Children Exposed to Domestic Violence

Collaborative Approaches to Intervention

Miriam Berkman, Robert L. Casey,
Steven J. Berkowitz, and Steven Marans

Police were called to the scene of a domestic disturbance. When officers arrived, they were greeted by a young woman who had a deep cut below one eye and bruises on her neck. Dishes and other household belongings were strewn about the apartment. A 7-year-old boy was silently watching TV in the living room. The woman reported that her live-in boyfriend had come home drunk, accused her of cheating on him, and had physically attacked her when she refused to talk about it. When he began to strangle her, the child had called 911. Officers called for emergency medical services, obtained a description of the boyfriend, and began a search of the neighborhood.

This case represents just one of the hundreds of thousands of episodes each year in which police officers come into contact with children affected by domestic violence. For most police officers, children present at scenes of domestic violence tend to be invisible, and law enforcement interventions revolve around the arrest and prosecution of adult offenders, often coupled with social service referral for adult victims. For children and families, however, contact with the police can present not only a moment of tragedy but also an opportunity for adults to recognize the children's experience and to intervene before children suffer serious disruptions of development.

INCIDENCE OF POLICE CONTACT

Precise nationwide data regarding police contacts with child witnesses of domestic violence are unavailable because existing criminal justice statistics report rates of arrests by type of crime. Ordinarily, these data do not include information regarding the nature of the relationship between victim and offender or the presence of child witnesses. Some states do maintain statistics regarding criminal reports of domestic violence, though each jurisdiction uses its own definition of the crimes included. For example, police departments throughout the state of Connecticut reported 20,927 arrests for family violence in 2001, with children present in 43% of the cases (Connecticut Department of Public Safety, 2002). In New Haven, Connecticut, a small city of approximately 110,000 people, police investigate an average of 2,000 domestic violence incidents a year; children are noted to be present in 55% of police reports (New Haven Department of Public Service, personal communication). In the Spousal Assault Replication Project (SARP), a five-city study of police responses to domestic violence, households with children were more likely to report an incident of domestic violence than households without children. Children under 5 years old were more likely than older children to witness violence within their homes, and were more likely to witness multiple episodes of domestic violence (Fantuzzo, Boruch, Beriama, & Atkins, 1997). It is also well known and documented that domestic violence is greatly underreported to the police (see, e.g., Tjaden & Thoennes, 2000), and so the actual number of children who witness violence against their caregivers is much higher than the numbers reported to the police. Chapter 2 provides information about the estimated number of children exposed to domestic violence.

THE POLICE PERSPECTIVE ON EFFECTS
OF VIOLENCE ON CHILDREN

Chapter 3 documents the range of risks and problems that children experience as a consequence of their exposure to domestic violence, including increases in aggression, oppositional behavior, depression, anxiety, as well as decreases in school achievement. Police officers know from experience that the children they encounter at scenes of domestic violence are often visibly distressed. They appear frightened, sad, or angry. Sometimes they look vacant or numb. Children may respond to officers by begging them not to leave, by berating them for arresting a violent but loved parent, or by ignoring the officers' presence. Officers may hear reports from parents that their children refuse to go to school, have trouble sleeping, or constantly fight with siblings and classmates.

From the perspective of police officers, one of the most easily observable and distressing consequences of children's exposure to domestic violence is the increased likelihood that the child will become involved in violence, either as a victim or as an aggressor. Police are well acquainted with the experience of seeing a child first as a passive witness to his or her parents' fights and later arresting the same child for adolescent delinquency. Both arrestees and victims in domestic violence cases frequently report histories of repeatedly witnessing similar abuse between their own parents or caregivers.

THE FRUSTRATION OF DEALING WITH DOMESTIC VIOLENCE CASES

It is often frustrating for police officers to deal with cases of domestic violence. Some victims may resist the officer's efforts to help them, either by refusing to provide the information that would allow the officer to make an arrest or by minimizing the extent of the violence so as to limit the officer's ability to substantiate serious charges. Other victims may initially cooperate actively with the criminal investigation, only to change their minds and bail the defendant out of jail or appear in court requesting that charges be dropped. Even when the victim herself wishes to hold her aggressive partner criminally responsible, she may be so overwhelmed and emotional that she has difficulty providing the officer with the specific information needed to make an arrest on charges appropriate to the seriousness of the incident.

Criminal justice remedies also tend to be limited. Most calls for police service in domestic violence cases concern misdemeanor offenses, such as breach of the peace, threatening, and simple assault, which do not carry significant penalties and rarely justify lengthy pretrial detention. It is not unusual for defendants to be released within days, if not hours, with court orders of protection that may be worth little more than the paper they are written on. In this context, officers frequently find themselves responding repeatedly to the same addresses, with little expectation that their attempts to intervene will result in any real change.

THE ROLE OF THE POLICE IN CASES
OF DOMESTIC VIOLENCE

Domestic violence calls present police with highly charged emotional situations that can be dangerous to everyone involved. The personal and emotional nature of the calls can also arouse strong feelings in the responding officers, particularly if they remind officers of similar circumstances in their own family or friendship network. It is not easy to remain neutral and professional in the face of such physical and emotional stimuli, and the temptation may be great either to overreact to one party or the other or to move on to the next call as quickly as possible. As both first responders and societal figures of authority, police officers are in a unique position to intervene in the lives of children who are exposed to violence in their homes (Marans, Berkman, & Cohen, 1996). Though the specific event that prompts a police response is rarely the first incident of violence in the family, officers may be the abused woman's first point of contact with a network of social institutions that may provide greater safety and support for herself and her children. This chapter will describe the efforts of one city's police, abused women's advocates, and mental health clinicians to develop new ways of working together to increase the safety and security of abused women and their children.

THE CHILD DEVELOPMENT
COMMUNITY POLICING PROGRAM

The Child Development Community Policing Program (CD-CP) was established in 1991 as an innovative collaboration between the Yale University Child Study Center (CSC) and the New Haven Department of Police Service (NHDPS) (Marans & Adnopoz, 1995; Marans, Berkowitz, & Cohen, 1998; Marans & Cohen, 1993; Marans, Murphy, & Berkowitz, 2002). The partnership had its foundation in the transition of the New Haven police to a philosophy of community-based policing in which the need to arrest offenders is integrated with a preventive approach based on relationships and problem-solving efforts with a range of community constituencies. As the model brings police officers into regular, ongoing contact with children and families within a given neighborhood, it requires a new type of police officer with specialized training, supervision, and support.

The CD-CP program developed out of the joint recognition that police officers and mental health clinicians share serious concerns about the fate of children and families exposed to violence in their homes and in the larger community. Though police officers come into daily contact with children who are victims, witnesses, and perpetrators of violence, they do not have the professional expertise, the time, or the resources to meet these children's psychological needs. Conversely, clinic-based mental health professionals may be professionally equipped to respond to children's psychological distress following episodes of violence; however, the acutely traumatized children who are most in need of clinical service are rarely seen in existing outpatient clinics until months or years later, when chronic symptoms bring them to the attention of parents, teachers, or the juvenile courts. By bringing together the different perspectives of law enforcement and child development and advocacy, the CD-CP collaboration provides an opportunity for a more comprehensive understanding of the impact of violence on children and families.

Description of the Program

When the CD-CP program began, it was defined as a partnership between police officers and mental health clinicians. Over the past 10 years, the partnership has expanded to become a more comprehensive collaboration among police, mental health clinicians, juvenile justice professionals, abused women's advocates, child protective services, and other community workers. The program focuses on:

- Improving police and mental health responses to violence exposure and potential trauma.
- Increasing children's sense of safety and security.
- Improving the police–community relationship.
- Decreasing children's maladaptive responses following exposure to violence.

The CD-CP program consists of several interrelated training and service components that promote the development of a shared frame of reference, close working relationships, and exchange of information between professionals responding collaboratively to children and families victimized by violence. These include the following:

Child Development Training for Police Officers and Other Professionals

Police officers, abused women's advocates, clinicians, probation officers, and child protection workers receive training in basic principles of child development and their application to child-oriented community interventions. Increased knowledge about children's development and the potential impact of trauma allows police, probation, and other professionals to take children's needs into account as they do their work.

Police Training for Clinicians

Clinicians participate in a related fellowship designed to familiarize them with community policing and law enforcement strategies. Clinicians learn about police roles in the community and protocols for police practice through seminars and regular observational "ride alongs" with patrol officers. Greater familiarity with the potential uses and limitations of police authority expands clinicians' options in designing and implementing effective intervention strategies.

Twenty-Four-Hour Consultation Service

A key component of the CD-CP program is a 24-hour consultation service staffed by mental health clinicians and advocates who are available to respond immediately to police requests for consultation and intervention with children and families exposed to violence. Clinicians provide immediate intervention for children who otherwise might not be identified for mental health services, as well as consultation to officers regarding their own responses to children and families.

Weekly Program Conference

Clinicians, officers, and other collaborators discuss cases referred to the consultation service during a weekly program conference to develop, review, and evaluate planned responses. The program conference fosters consistent and open relationships across disciplines and provides a forum for discussing systemic and organizational issues that may interfere with effective intervention on behalf of children exposed to violence.

The Effects of the Program

The CD-CP program has had a profound effect on police policy and practice in New Haven, as demonstrated by the following:

- Before the establishment of the CD-CP, police had not referred any children for clinical services. From 1995 to the present, clinicians receive an average of 10 referrals or requests for consultations per week.

- All new police recruits and all supervisory officers receive a 1-day course in developmental issues for children.
- There is a police officer either assigned to or responsible for every New Haven public school.
- CD-CP clinicians' names and pager numbers are listed at every dispatch station in the police department's central communications unit.
- The CD-CP clinician is listed as an essential contact in the police department's formal notification system for serious events. Since 1998, the police reporting form requires that all children present at a crime scene be listed, and there is a checkoff box for contact with a CD-CP clinician.

Case Examples

The following cases illustrate the CD-CP model of coordinated police–mental health intervention in responding immediately to children who witness domestic violence. In the first case, police officers assumed the primary personal contact with the children. The consulting clinician assisted officers in tailoring their responses to the developmental needs of the children and provided information and acute support to the adults responsible for the children's care. In this case, as with many others in the program's experience, intervention was limited to the acute collaborative response.

Acute Collaborative Response

Police were called to a domestic disturbance. A man had stabbed a woman with a meat cleaver in the presence of their two children, ages 2 and 8. When police arrived, they found the adults still arguing and the children curled up on the couch, splattered with blood. Officers arranged for the woman to be transported to the hospital by ambulance and arrested the man. Police called Child Protective Services and transported the children to police headquarters. They also called the CD-CP clinician on call and the children's grandmother, and requested that both also respond to the police station. Officers understood that the best thing they could do to help these children regain a sense of safety and security was to arrange for them to be cared for by a trusted and familiar adult, and so they did not wait for CPS but called the grandmother immediately.

At the police station, officers brought the children food and found a comfortable, quiet place for them to wait for their grandmother, the clinician, and CPS. As they waited, the 2-year-old,

Erica, complained that she "had blood on her" and became agitated that it would not come off. In consultation with the on-call clinician, officers helped Erica wash the blood from her hands and provided her with a clean shirt. This stopped the child from being visually confronted with a powerful reminder of the overwhelming incident. An officer then held Erica in his lap and let her fall asleep. Meanwhile, other officers worked closely with CPS to investigate the safety and appropriateness of the children's grandmother as a temporary guardian.

Upon arrival at the police station, the 8-year-old, Sarah, cried inconsolably, but she began to regain her composure as she greedily devoured the food provided by the officers. One officer sat next to her as she ate, and she began to recount the details of the incident she had witnessed. One striking feature of Sarah's story was that she stated several times that she could have stopped them from fighting if only she had gotten the baseball bat from the closet and threatened to hit her stepfather. She also asked repeatedly what was going to happen to her mother and stepfather. She was concerned that she would never see them again.

The officer understood that Sarah's wishes to have heroically stopped the fighting were an expression of her attempt to avoid feeling so helpless and small. He therefore responded by emphasizing the action she did take and told her, "I know you wish that things were different, but you did the right thing by keeping yourself and your sister safe." In consultation with the clinician, the officer also provided honest answers to Sarah's questions about her parents. The officer obtained a medical status report from the hospital, and told Sarah her mother was being treated and would most likely be returning home the next day. He also told her that her stepfather was arrested and was staying in jail for the night because what he had done was dangerous and against the law. A judge would see him in the morning and decide when he could come home. Although it was difficult for the officers to discuss such unpleasant issues with a young child, they understood that it was better to tell the truth than to leave the questions unanswered and allow the child to imagine facts even worse than reality.

Eventually, CPS approved the grandmother as temporary guardian, and she took the children home. Before she left, the clinician met with her to discuss the reactions she might expect from both children and the ways in which she could best support them. The clinician also offered follow-up meetings with the children and family. On telephone follow-up a few days later, the mother had been discharged from the hospital. She reported the children were doing fine, and there was no further clinical contact. Neighborhood officers made several unscheduled follow-up visits to the home to check on the mother's safety and the children's reactions. The mother reported being grateful for the officers' support, but declined referrals for any additional services. There have been no further calls for police services to the address.

In this case, well-trained officers, aided by the on-call clinician, were able to provide immediate support to the children and their grandmother at the moment of acute crisis. The immediate intervention focused on the children's developmental needs for stability and familiarity, as well as age-appropriate information to correct misperceptions and diminish the anxiety fueled by imagination. The team provided support and information for the children's caregivers to assist them in providing the necessary support and nurturance for the children.

In other CD-CP cases, police contact with children and families in an acute moment of crisis provides a link to ongoing clinical treatment for children and adults. Officers facilitate parents' engagement with clinicians by respectfully communicating their concerns for the children's vulnerability and by making services accessible. Once a parent accepts a clinical referral, the police–mental health collaboration is not over. Rather, clinicians and officers maintain contact as needed and as permitted by the family to maximize safety and security. The following case presents an example of acute response leading to extended treatment and collaborative intervention.

Acute Response Followed by Extensive Clinical Intervention

Jean and her boyfriend were driving to dinner when they happened to drive past Jean's ex-husband Bill. Bill was taking their sons, Billy (age 10) and Michael (age 8), to the movies. Bill had heard rumors that his ex-wife was seeing someone, but he was not certain it was true until he saw her in the car. He quickly turned his car around and began to follow Jean's car as closely as traffic would allow, cursing and yelling despite the presence of his sons in the backseat. He drove up onto the sidewalk, nearly hitting several pedestrians, and cut in front of Jean's car. Both boys sat in the backseat, terrified and crying. Jean jumped out of her boyfriend's car to comfort her boys through an open car window. Bill then reached over and punched her in the face, bloodying her nose. Jean's companion witnessed the assault and called the police on his car phone. By the time the police arrived, Bill had fled back to his house, where he was later arrested, and the boys were returned to the care of their mother.

Although Jean had initially declined clinical services offered by the police, the responding officers were extremely concerned about the children and paged the on-call clinician for a consultation. An officer spoke with the clinician on the phone while Jean listened. The officer described the details of the incident, expressed concern for the children, and asked questions about how he might be helpful to the boys at that moment. He began to include Jean in the discussion by asking her questions about the children. The officer served as a go-between until he sensed that Jean was willing to speak directly with the clinician, at which point he offered her the phone. Jean agreed to have the boys evaluated the next day. The officer understood that Jean needed to be in charge of making decisions for her children and that it would do no good either to lecture her on why she should accept the offer of immediate services or to walk away feeling frustrated and angry with her. By demonstrating patience, respect, and genuine concern, the responding officers successfully brokered the referral.

During the evaluation, both boys expressed their confusion and conflicted loyalty about what had happened the night before and throughout their parents' breakup. While they were angry with their father for hitting their mother, they also felt betrayed by their mother for leaving their father and dating another man. The boys revealed that their father had pressured them to spy on their mother and would frequently question them about Jean's whereabouts, her friends, and any phone calls she received.

Both children continued in weekly psychotherapy, and the children's therapist also met separately with each of the parents in an attempt to help them to understand the difficulties facing their boys. In particular, the therapist urged Bill to shelter his sons from the animosity between the adults and to stop having them spy on their mother. Bill vowed that he would protect the boys from his anger and sadness. Despite this promise and a "no contact" order issued by the court, Bill forced his older son to deliver a threatening note. Billy was devastated when his mother read the note and immediately burst into tears.

The treating clinician met with Jean and then facilitated a meeting about the violation between Jean, her advocate, and domestic violence detectives. Jean reluctantly concluded that further police action was likely the only way to contain Bill's behavior. However, she found it extremely difficult emotionally to seek Bill's arrest because she knew the boys loved their father and she did not want to feel responsible for interfering with their relationship with him. With substantial support from the boys' therapist, her advocate, and police detectives, Jean did provide a statement detailing Bill's violations of the court order. Bill was arrested for the second time with the message that further disregard for court orders and the well-being of his children would not be tolerated. To date, Bill has been able to contain his behavior.

This case provides an example of the essential ongoing connection between legal and therapeutic interventions. As the children's therapist became increasingly aware of the detrimental effects on them of their father's repeated violation of the court order, the therapist supported the mother to take legal action to protect her children. The therapist understood that without a cessation of the father's actions, therapy was futile. As the therapist helped Jean to understand the experience from the children's perspective and to see that they needed her active protection, she was able to exercise her legal rights on their behalf.

THE CD-CP DOMESTIC VIOLENCE
INTERVENTION PROJECT

Since the inception of the CD-CP Program, approximately 30% of the calls received through the consultation service have concerned children and adolescents who have witnessed violence against their mothers by an intimate partner. A specialty team was developed within CD-CP, beginning in 1998, with the support of the U.S. Department of Justice Violence Against Women Office, to develop responses more specifically tailored to the needs of abused women.

The CD-CP Domestic Violence Intervention Project combines acute clinical response with coordinated follow-up by clinicians, outreach workers, neighborhood patrol officers, domestic violence detectives, and domestic violence advocates. The intervention project uses the basic principles of the CD-CP program, including the immediate identification of children and families exposed to violence, multidisciplinary collaborative approaches to address the impact of violence, as well as coordinated intervention and intensive case management. The Domestic Violence Intervention Project expands the CD-CP approach by establishing closer linkages with domestic violence advocates and court personnel and intensifying the role of neighborhood police in monitoring the safety of abused women and their children. Cases are referred to the team by police officers, using the CD-CP 24-hour on-call service for immediate intervention, or by domestic violence advocates who recognize a need for clinical intervention through contact with victims in the specialized domestic violence court.

In addition, the team has implemented a neighborhood-based home visit follow-up project in 2 out of 10 policing districts within the city. In these pilot districts, detectives in the domestic violence unit identify households where an intimate partner assault has been reported. Police-advocate teams are then assigned to provide follow-up home visits. The visits are intended to monitor victim safety, improve understanding and enforcement of court orders, and increase parents' access to information and supportive services for themselves and their children. Outreach advocates, in consultation with staff clinicians, provide a safety assessment, attend to posttraumatic symptoms, facilitate engagement with mental health treatment or other social services, and assist in the development of plans designed to reduce subsequent violence. Neighborhood officers provide specific guidance in safety planning, assist in securing necessary court orders, and become a resource in the event of future emergencies (see Chapter 6 for a detailed discussion of safety planning). Court-based advocates assist families as they participate in complex or lengthy legal proceedings, and ensure that realistic legal options and court rulings are communicated. Assigning neighborhood officers to initiate contact with victims and their children outside of the moment of violent crisis sets a tone within the community that police give high priority to addressing domestic violence, particularly when children are involved. By reaching out to victims of domestic violence on the basis of concern for the impact violence has on their children, the project capitalizes on mothers' investment in their children's well-being, which is hypothesized to be a prime motivation for seeking greater safety. The project team engages women in addressing complex problems by first emphasizing that children's most basic emotional need is consistent parental care within an environment of physical safety. The team then works with the mother to attend to the combination of practical and psychological issues that affect safety and consistency.

Case Examples

Two examples drawn from the early experience of the home visit project team illustrate some of the ways in which the outreach visits can enhance victims' safety and security. In the first case, neighborhood patrol officers, detectives, advocates, and consulting clinicians employed frequent home visits to monitor the victim's immediate safety while simultaneously expediting confinement of a dangerous defendant.

Follow-Up Visits as Part of Intensive Law Enforcement and Safety Planning

The neighborhood patrol/advocacy follow-up team received a request from the Domestic Violence Unit supervisor to make a home visit and check the safety of Jessica, a 14-year-old girl. The case had been assigned to the team because there had been two calls for police service within the previous week related to drug abuse and suicide and homicide threats by Jessica's former boyfriend, Alan, age 16. After consultation with clinical members of the CD-CP Domestic Violence Team, the DVU supervisor was concerned about the high risk of repeat violence presented by Alan. The team agreed to assign the case for home visit monitoring of the victim's safety, to expedite processing of all outstanding warrants, and to coordinate psychiatric response through the CD-CP on-call clinical service.

The first call to police had come from Jessica's mother. She reported that Alan had appeared at Jessica's home, screaming outside her window and demanding to talk to her. Jessica's mother told him to leave, and he then proceeded to throw both a rock and a knife at the windows, breaking one and damaging the other. Responding officers could not locate and arrest Alan that night, and applied for an arrest warrant. The following night, police were dispatched to Alan's home in response to a complaint from his mother. Responding officers found him making suicidal and homicidal remarks and also smelling of alcohol and crack cocaine. Police transported Alan to the local hospital, where he was briefly admitted to the psychiatric ward. He was discharged as soon as he was no longer acutely suicidal.

A neighborhood patrol officer and outreach advocate visited Jessica and her family. They heard how frightened Jessica was, as well as her report that Alan had made new threats against her from a telephone in the psychiatric unit. The team obtained a 911-programmed cell phone for Jessica to have with her at all times and arranged for a detective to install an emergency notification system in her home the following day. This would allow any member of the family to place an immediate call to the police by pressing a panic button. The team gave Jessica and her mother telephone and pager numbers to reach police and advocates at any time to obtain assistance or to give new information about Alan. The team also made plans for frequent repeat visits until Alan was arrested.

A few days later, Alan's mother again called the police because he was threatening to kill himself. Again, he was taken to the hospital. The supervisor in charge of the Police Department's Domestic Violence Unit, in consultation with the CD-CP program's on-call psychiatrist, contacted the hospital and provided additional essential information to justify Alan's admission for several days, rather than just overnight as before. The DVU supervisor also arranged for the hospital staff to notify her personally prior to Alan's discharge. While Alan was hospitalized, the DVU supervisor made sure that the warrant for his arrest was expedited so that he would move directly from hospital to detention and Jessica's safety would be maintained. When police were notified of Alan's discharge from the hospital, two detectives waited outside his home to arrest him. The prosecutor had been notified and requested a high pretrial bond. Eventually, Alan pleaded guilty and was placed on probation, with a special condition that he stay away from Jessica.

In this case, police, mental health professionals, and advocates worked closely together to identify the high risk posed by the defendant and to confine him through a combination of psychiatric and criminal processes. The team provided additional security to support the teenage victim through personal home visits and communication technology.

Advocates and officers involved in the neighborhood home visit project report that one frequent outcome of the visits is that victims achieve a greater understanding of their rights within the legal system, particularly with respect to the meaning of court orders of protection. Abused women's increased appreciation of their rights and options supports greater autonomy in their decision making for themselves and for their children. The following case describes an example in which the outreach visit brought information and policing support to a woman who would not have otherwise contacted the police.

Home Visit Clarifies Court Orders and Results in Arrest of Defendant

The neighborhood patrol home visit project received a request to visit the home of Tamika, a 20-year-old mother of two children (ages 2 and 1). Four days previously, Tamika's boyfriend, Charles, had assaulted her, ripped the phone off the wall, and ripped her necklace off her neck. Charles was arrested at the scene. Responding officers did not call the CD-CP pager service, perhaps because the children were so young, it was very late at night, or the police shift was very busy. On the first home visit by the team, Charles was present and in violation of a court order issued at his arraignment requiring that he vacate the home and have no contact with Tamika. Charles was placed under arrest without incident. Tamika was surprised and very grateful that Charles was removed. She had not reported his presence to police or court-based advocates because he had told her that this was his residence and so he was allowed to be there. The team made several additional home visits to monitor Tamika's continued safety and Charles's compliance with the court order. The advocate provided Tamika with information about young children's common responses to violence and encouraged her to call if she had any further questions or needs.

Approximately 1 month later, Tamika contacted the advocate regarding an eviction notice that she had received. From scanning the police reports, the public housing manager found that, at the time of the incident, Charles had been living with her, contrary to the provisions of her lease. The advocate accompanied Tamika to a meeting with the housing manager, where they explained Tamika's situation and had Charles's name added to the Housing Authority's official trespass list for that complex.

The following month, upon Charles's release from jail, he was once again in the housing complex loitering near Tamika's apartment. Tamika called the advocate, who urged her to call the police. Tamika was afraid she would herself be arrested or that Charles would know she had called the police, and she feared retaliation from Charles or his friends. With Tamika's permission, the advocate called the police substation and asked that a patrol officer drive through the complex as if on routine patrol; however, the officer did not see Charles. The next evening the advocate made an additional home visit with an officer, who explained to Tamika the conditions under which Charles could be arrested, emphasized that she could not be arrested for reporting him, and encouraged her to call the police herself the next time that he trespassed. The officer also encouraged her to call the property manager so that the officers assigned to the complex were aware of his trespassing.

In this case, the unscheduled home visit by the police/advocate team resulted in arrest of the defendant for violation of a criminal protective order. The violation would likely never have come to light otherwise because Tamika did not understand her rights under the order. Strict enforcement of the court's orders through cooperation between neighborhood officers, housing managers, CD-CP advocates, and court personnel facilitated Tamika's safety and separation from Charles.

PRELIMINARY PROGRAM EVALUATION DATA

Preliminary comparisons of victims receiving the police/advocate intervention (intervention group) with a group of victims who did not (comparison group), suggest a decrease in the number of repeat calls for police service by the intervention group for the year following the police/advocate home visit. A pilot group of 45 victims who received home visits during the first 6 months of the project was compared with 45 victims who did not receive the intervention. During the year following the visits, police received 11 calls from the intervention group regarding new incidents of domestic violence and 24 calls from the comparison group reporting new incidents. Although encouraging, this finding simply indicates that the intervention group did not call the police as often. It is not clear if this finding correlates with a decrease in violence. To better understand the impact of the intervention, a follow-up telephone survey was implemented, targeting victim satisfaction with the police/advocate home visit to determine whether the outreach visits deterred the victims from calling the police again. In the project's first year, 26% (54 victims) of the total intervention group (236 victims) have completed the survey, 2% refused (4 victims), and 60% (144 victims) were never reached despite multiple attempts. Of relevance, 94% of those who completed the survey stated that it was very easy or somewhat easy to speak with the police officer, 96% stated that it was very easy or somewhat easy to speak with the advocate, 74% stated that they felt an increase in their safety because of the police/advocate home visit (25% reported no change in their feelings of safety), and 91% found the visit to be helpful. Related to the decrease in calls-for-service for the intervention group, 86% responded that they would be more likely to call the police in the future as a result of the home visit. While far from conclusive, these preliminary data suggest that the reduction in repeat calls to the police is not likely to be the result of increased inhibition on the part of the victims.

SUMMARY AND CONCLUSIONS

As the New Haven CD-CP program demonstrates, police–mental health collaborations may have profound effects on the ways in which police officers deliver routine police services and also on the ways in which officers conceptualize their own roles in the lives of children and families. The police partnership with mental health professionals and abused women's advocates reflects a commitment to a philosophy of policing that addresses criminal activity in a social context rather than in a perspective limited to individual incidents. This change in perspective reorders police priorities and challenges officers to expand their field of vision and their repertoire of intervention strategies. An expanded perspective on policing can also include greater appreciation for the psychological role that well-trained and developmentally informed police can play in the lives of children and families.

Unlike other professionals, police officers respond to the scene immediately and are therefore present during the acute moment of crisis or soon after. As a result, police officers have unique opportunities to intervene at a time when many parents and children may be most receptive to accepting assistance because they are so acutely overwhelmed. In these moments, officers can provide a voice of reality that confirms for children and adults that something very serious and wrong did in fact take place. Police officers can support the child's caregiver in beginning to evaluate and plan for her own safety. In the immediate aftermath of a violent incident, officers can provide valuable information to the victim regarding the status of the offender, the likely conduct of court proceedings, and the existence of supportive services in the community. Officers can also act as brokers of social services. In these situations, officers not only provide information as a courtesy but also use their immediate presence and authoritative role to create a bridge between acute law enforcement response and longer-term problem solving.

In the ordinary course of their response to calls, police officers come into contact frequently with children exposed to and affected by domestic violence. These contacts present windows of opportunity for early identification of children who may be at risk for a host of developmental difficulties and opportunities to forge alliances with parents who may be struggling to meet their children's needs for safety and consistency. For officers, partnership with advocates, clinicians, and other professionals increases their ability to recognize the needs of vulnerable children, to develop more effective interventions, and to sustain their own attention to the complex and painful experience of abused women and their children. Coordinated intervention approaches, which capitalize on the unique authoritative role of the police, provide promising new strategies for interrupting the intergenerational cycle of violence.

REFERENCES

Connecticut Department of Public Safety. (2002, Spring). 2001 preliminary family violence report: Family violence reporting program. *Department of Public Safety, Connecticut State Police,* pp. 1–5.

Fantuzzo, J., Boruch, R., Beriama, A., & Atkins, M. (1997). Domestic violence and children: Prevalence and risk in five major U.S. cities. *Journal of the American Academy of Child and Adolescent Psychiatry, 36*(1), 116–122.

Marans, S., & Adnopoz, J. (1995). *The police–mental health partnership: A community-based response to urban violence.* New Haven, CT: Yale University Press.

Marans, S., Berkman, M., & Cohen, D. J. (1996) Child development and adaptation to catastrophic circumstances. In R. J. Apfel and B. Simon (Eds.), *Minefields in their hearts: The mental health of children in war and communal violence* (pp. 104–127). New Haven: Yale University Press.

Marans, S., Berkowitz, S. J., & Cohen, D. J. (1998). Police and mental health professionals: Collaborative responses to the impact of violence on children and families. *Child and Adolescent Psychiatric Clinics of North America, 7*(3), 635–651.

Marans, S., & Cohen, D. J. (1993). Children and inner-city violence: Strategies for intervention. In L. A. Leavitt & N. A. Fox (Eds.), *The psychological effects of war and violence on children* (pp. 281–301). Hillsdale, NJ: Erlbaum.

Marans, S., Murphy, R. A., & Berkowitz, S. J. (2002). Police–mental health responses to children exposed to violence: The Child Development Community Policing Program. In M. Lewis (Ed.), *Comprehensive textbook of child and adolescent psychiatry.* Baltimore, MD: Williams & Wilkins.

Tjaden, P. G., & Thoennes, N. (2000). *Extent, nature, and consequences of intimate partner violence.* Washington, DC: U.S. Department of Justice, Office of Justice Programs, National Institute of Justice.

11

The Role of Family Courts in Domestic Violence

The Canadian Experience

MARTHA SHAFFER and NICHOLAS BALA

During the past decade and a half there has been a dramatic increase in awareness within the justice system of the problem of wife abuse. While there is a need for much more research in this area, there is a growing body of social science research on wife abuse and its effects on children (see Chapter 2 for a detailed discussion). Some of this research is being translated into policy and is being reflected in judicial decisions. For example, many jurisdictions have adopted "mandatory charge/no drop" policies for the prosecution of domestic violence offenses. Increasingly, specialized criminal courts for prosecuting domestic violence cases are being established, with support services for victims and counseling programs for abusers. Wife abuse is a frequent topic at judicial education seminars and is included in police training. Professional schools in medicine, nursing, and law are increasingly including wife abuse in their curricula. These developments may be having some impact on wife abuse, as there is some evidence that rates of abuse in Canada may be slowly declining (Statistics Canada, 2001). Nonetheless, rates of spousal abuse remain unacceptably high and exact an enormous human and societal toll. While some progress is evident, the justice system often fails to protect or provide safety to abused women and their children. Nowhere is this more evident than in the context of family law cases, particularly those involving decisions about custody and access.[1] Although for the most part Canadian judges are aware that granting *custody* of a child to an abusive spouse is not in the child's best interests, courts routinely grant abusive spouses *unsupervised access* to their children. This situation cannot be attributed solely to judicial failure to appreciate the potential harms of unsupervised access. It is also brought about because other key players in the family law system, most notably mediators and lawyers, fail to advocate vigorously for their clients, assuming that access will be granted in almost all cases.

In this chapter, we examine 42 Canadian custody and access decisions over a 3½-year period in cases in which allegations of wife abuse were made. During the late 1980s and early 1990s, the attitude prevalent in the justice system, and in Canadian society more broadly, was that wife abuse was not relevant to custody or access. However, our review of decisions in the 1997–2000 period reveals that courts are generally showing an increasing sensitivity (Shaffer, in press). For the most part, courts appear to be aware of the dangers of awarding custody to abusive spouses, with the result that such awards are rare. While this is clearly a positive development for abused women and their children, the cases also suggest reasons to be concerned about the treatment of wife abuse in the family law system.

One source of concern is that the key players in the family justice system—lawyers, assessors, and judges—may be working with a simplistic notion of wife abuse that impairs their ability to "see" abuse in some cases. Another is that many, if not most, lawyers, assessors, and judges assume that contact with both parents is (almost) always in the child's best interests, in the absence of strong evidence that a parent has directly physically or sexually abused a child. This belief, as well as the idea that fathers have a "right" to see their children, appears to account for the routine use of unsupervised access awards, even in situations where a cessation of access or supervised access may be warranted.

THE STUDY

Our research into custody and access awards in cases involving wife abuse grew out of the concern that, as recently as a decade ago, many

Canadian judges did not regard even substantiated woman abuse as a relevant consideration in custody and access determinations (Canadian Panel on Violence Against Women, 1993). This approach to wife abuse is graphically illustrated by the 1988 Nova Scotia case of *Peterson v. Peterson* (1988). In *Peterson*, Judge Freeman (who has since been promoted to the Nova Scotia Court of Appeal) awarded interim custody of two young children to their father, despite evidence that he had abused his wife during their 8-year marriage. There was also evidence that Mr. Peterson had struck the older child, who was seven at the time of parental separation, on at least two occasions. When the child's aunt intervened on the first occasion to try to protect the child, Mr. Peterson drove her head through a wall, causing the aunt to suffer a black eye and facial swelling. In the second incident, the father became angry with the boy and kicked him in the chest. At the end of the marriage, upon discovering that Mrs. Peterson had taken a lover, Mr. Peterson severely assaulted Mrs. Peterson and her lover using a metal bar. After the assault, while Mrs. Peterson lay naked and bleeding on the floor, Mr. Peterson brought their 7-year-old to the door of the room and told him to look at his mother.

The court accepted that Mr. Peterson had a predisposition to violence and exhibited a lack of "parental wisdom" in deliberately exposing his son to Mrs. Peterson's "anguish and humiliation." It also accepted that Mrs. Peterson had been the primary caregiver for the children and was "an excellent mother." Nonetheless, the court awarded interim custody to Mr. Peterson, emphasizing the importance to the children of having "the stabilizing factor of continuing to live in the home they are used to, with all persons of importance in their lives, excepting their mother, in the relationship they have always known." Perhaps most inexplicably, the judge observed that "there was no evidence of intolerable cruelty" on Mr. Peterson's part, as "his conduct had been tolerated by Marlene Peterson through eight years of marriage and two children." Despite accepting the evidence of Mr. Peterson's violence, in the court's view, Mrs. Peterson bore "primary responsibility" for the breakup of marriage and the termination of the children's "ideal lifestyle."

In minimizing the significance of abuse in the breakdown of the Peterson's marriage and awarding custody to a man with a long history of abusive conduct toward his wife and children, the court in the *Peterson* case reflected many of the deeply troubling attitudes about wife abuse prevalent in the Canadian judiciary and among society more broadly at that time. The purpose of our research is to examine whether the judicial approach to the issue of wife abuse and its effect on custody and access decisions has changed. One would expect some changes: judicial education programs should have increased judicial knowledge on the subject, including some knowledge about the emerging body of psychological research on the impact on children of exposure to wife abuse. The composition of the Canadian judiciary has also changed in the past decade and a half, with more women judges being appointed, and this too may have an impact on judicial approaches to wife abuse.

Method

We examined all Canadian cases reported on Quicklaw, a computer database of legal decisions, over a 3½-year period from January 1997 to May 2000, in which the terms "spouse abuse" or "wife abuse" and "custody" or "access" appeared. In examining these cases, we sought to get a sense of how judges approached the issue of wife abuse in the custody and access context. Did judges tend to take women's claims seriously, or did they view them as strategic ploys to buttress their custody claims? Did judges continue to award custody to abusive men? What kinds of access awards were made to men who have abused their intimate female partner?

Our search generated 42 cases in which allegations of spousal abuse had been made in custody or access disputes, a small number in light of the number of cases throughout Canada in which wife abuse would have been an issue over a 3½-year period. Our search would have missed cases in which the court did not use one of our search terms (for example, where a court referred to abuse but did not use the term "wife" or "spousal") or cases in which the court rendered oral, rather than written, reasons. Although the small sample size makes it difficult to determine how representative these cases are of all cases in which abusive men made custody or access claims, our results are largely consistent with those found by a New Brunswick research team that conducted a much broader study of reported and unreported judicial decisions in that province (Neilson et. al., 2001).

Analysis of the Cases

Our analysis of these cases suggests there is both cause for optimism as well as reason for concern. The optimism stems from the fact that judges appear to be much more cognizant than in the past that awarding custody to an abusive man is not in a child's best interests. Courts frequently stated that wife abuse is harmful to children and therefore falls in the category of conduct courts can legitimately consider in custody disputes, conduct that is relevant to a person's ability to act as a parent. Such statements were not prominent among cases decided as recently as 10 years ago. Perhaps more importantly, in terms of results, judges rarely granted custody to a man who abused his partner *provided* they accepted the woman's claims of abuse as valid. The court accepted the allegations in 31 of the 42 cases; of those 31, the mother received custody in 28, the father in 1, and joint custody was ordered in 2 cases.

However, our research reveals three areas of continuing concern:

- We found problematic statements about spousal violence, and questionable approaches to the allegations of wife abuse in some cases. Some judges may have simplistic notions of wife abuse, making them unable to "see" abuse that does not conform to the stereotypical "abused woman."
- There is a problem with the training of assessors, usually mental health professionals who, at the request of the court or with the consent of both parties, interview parents, children, and other relevant people and offer suggestions to the court of the best plan for the children. It appears that some assessors have little understanding of wife abuse and its impact on children.
- Access orders are a significant source of problems, as they often place women and their children at risk.

PROBLEMATIC JUDICIAL ATTITUDES AND APPROACHES

In our observation, the most significant changes in judicial approaches to wife abuse are in cases where the abuse takes the form of severe physical violence well documented by police or medical reports. Not only do judges accept that awarding custody to the abuser is not in the children's best interests in these cases, they also seem to have a good understanding of the dynamics of the relationships involving obviously "abused" women. Thus, in these cases, courts are quick to reject claims of self-defense made by men, noting that the disparity in size and strength between the spouses makes these claims not credible. Courts also frequently noted that husbands seemed more concerned with "winning" the custody dispute than with their children's best interests.

There are, however, concerns that the courts have greater difficulty dealing with abuse claims where the violence has been less extreme, where the woman has not been a passive victim, or where the violence is either poorly documented or not documented at all. In 11 of the 42 cases in our sample, courts found the woman's abuse allegations to be exaggerated (6 cases) or unfounded (5 cases). In most of these cases, it was difficult to assess the validity of the court's conclusions because the judge did not provide detailed reasons for disbelieving the women's claims. It is possible that some of the women may have exaggerated or even fabricated their abuse allegations; stories are often embellished in the context of litigation. It is, however, also possible that judges may have failed to "see" the abuse, either because it was not documented or because it did not take a stereotypical form.

In the absence of such documentation as police reports, medical records, disclosures to family and friends, or witnesses to the abuse, some judges have difficulty finding that the abuse occurred. In part, this difficulty may arise from the legal requirement to prove allegations on a balance of probabilities. Where there are no witnesses or documentation, courts may find that women fail to meet this standard, especially when women give only a generalized account of abuse (see *V.(L.) v. B.(T.)*, 2000). The problem of proving abuse to the court's satisfaction is a longstanding one, despite the knowledge that women usually endure many episodes of violence before calling the police, and that when they seek medical attention they often give doctors false explanations for their injuries (Statistics Canada, 2000). Some lawyers even advise their female clients not to raise abuse where they do not have sufficient evidence to corroborate their claims, for fear of being seen as making false allegations (Nielson et al., 2001).

Problems of proof did not, however, seem to account for all of the cases in which courts found the woman's allegations of abuse to be exaggerated or unfounded. Some of the cases reveal that courts had difficulty accepting or appreciating abuse claims where the abuse was largely emotional or verbal. In these cases, courts may not even conceptualize the conduct as abusive, viewing it instead as mutual conflict or discord.

Courts may also fail to recognize relationships as abusive where both spouses have engaged in violent behavior, as these cases also depart from the stereotypical model of the "abused woman." Even though in many of these cases one spouse is the primary aggressor, courts may mischaracterize them as involving mutual abuse, suggesting that both spouses are equally responsible for the violence. Several cases in our sample were characterized as involving mutual abuse, but because the court did not provide details of the relationships, it was impossible to assess the accuracy of this characterization. For example, in *Cadeau v. Martell,* the court described the spouses as "mutually engaged in conflictual behavior resulting in physical altercations." The court came to this conclusion despite holding that it "could not, on the evidence, conclude that [the wife] engaged in physical violence" but that it could "conclude on the evidence that in this relationship and in his last marriage . . . the [husband] has engaged in domestic violence that was, by his description, a serious breach of the peace." The characterization of this relationship as one of mutual conflict may not have been appropriate, in light of the husband's history of violence and the fact that he had pled guilty in criminal court to an assault in which he placed his hands over his wife's mouth and around her neck.

The tendency to mischaracterize cases as involving mutual abuse is troubling because it may fail to recognize the power dynamics at work in many relationships (Dalton, 1999). It becomes even more problematic if custody reforms are enacted that create presumptions against awarding custody or unsupervised access to abusers. Presumptions of this type have been enacted in several jurisdictions in the United States (Lemon, 2001).

Finally, although these are the exceptions rather than the rule, in a small number of cases, courts still award custody or joint custody to men who have abused their wives. There were two cases in our sample in which abusive men received joint custody, with the result that women were forced to share parenting with their abusive former spouses. In one of these cases, M.(G.E.) v. M.(C.) (1999), the court's decision can be understood in the context of the mother requesting joint custody, with her having primary care and control, in opposition to her husband seeking sole custody. Although the court rejected the father's claim for sole custody, its decision to order joint custody is troubling in light of the judge's observations that "this is really an abuse case" and "Mr. G.E.M. has a severe anger problem and absent any treatment of this problem, I am fearful that the health, safety and indeed the best interests of the children could be placed at risk by Mr. G.E.M. gaining sole custody." At best, it is difficult to see how a joint custody order could adequately address these concerns for the children's safety. While the parents had previously agreed to an interim joint custody arrangement, research in both Canada and Australia demonstrates that women leaving abusive relationships frequently agree to joint custody and access conditions that they do not believe are safe for their children (Nielson et al., 2001; Bala et al., 1998; Rhoades, Graycar, & Harrison, 2000). This suggests that judges (as well as lawyers and mediators) should be prepared to reject proposals for joint custody arrangements that may pose dangers to women or children.

In the other case, Mbaruk v. Mbaruk (1997), the court awarded joint custody with the father having primary residence, in large part because the children had resided with the father for 16 months preceding the decision. The court made this order despite finding that the father was a "rigid and domineering person" who had physically abused the mother during the marriage and who continued to denigrate and demean her after separation, including in the courtroom. There was also evidence that the father was attempting to undermine the mother's relationship with the children by limiting her access and by encouraging them to act out against her. The court's decision in this case seems to place inordinate emphasis on the "status quo," a situation that developed because the mother had difficulty coping with parenting and workplace demands after extricating herself from an abusive relationship. The decision also fails to give adequate weight to the fact that the mother had recovered her emotional health and self-confidence by the time of the trial. In the result, the decision effectively rewarded a controlling and abusive father for undermining the mother's parenting abilities and relationship with her children.

Despite these two cases, our overall conclusion is that, for the most part, judges are taking claims of wife abuse seriously. Judges show the greatest responsiveness in cases with documented and fairly serious levels of physical violence, at least insofar as custody decisions are concerned. The courts have more difficulty with cases in which the violence is less well documented or where the pattern of abuse is not the stereotypical one of repeated physical battering, either because the abuse is predominantly emotional or verbal or because the woman has also used violence. In these cases, it is not clear whether judges are adequately analyzing the dynamics of the relationship or whether they are incorrectly dismissing women's claims as unfounded or as involving mutual abuse. This is significant because judges award both sole and joint custody to men in cases of "mutual abuse" and cases where the allegations are held to be unfounded. Proving abuse remains a challenge. Advocates for victims of spousal abuse, whether lawyers or in the social service field, must try to find as much evidence as they can to help prove that abuse occurred, recognizing that in the court system proof and credibility are often central issues.

INADEQUATE TRAINING OF ASSESSORS

Custody assessments can place abused women and children at risk if the assessor does not have a competent understanding of the impact on children of exposure to wife abuse and of the dynamics of abusive relationships. In several cases in our sample, assessors submitted reports that showed a flawed understanding of wife abuse issues, and which, if followed, could have endangered the physical safety or emotional well-being of children and their mothers. In *Mbaruk v. Mbaruk,* described in the previous section, the assessor "rejected any suggestion that violence or abuse in the marriage relationship could have an impact on the children" and recommended that a father with a history of spousal abuse should receive joint custody. Finding these views in a custody assessment completed in 1995 is disturbing enough; it is even more disturbing in light of the fact that the assessor was a Family Court Counselor. Even the judge questioned the value of this report, although he ultimately ordered joint custody.

Another clearly flawed assessment was presented to the court in the case of *M.(G.E.) v. M.(C.)*, also described in the preceding section. An assessor from Family Conciliation Services recommended that a man with a severe anger problem and a history of abuse have sole custody and the mother have access on alternate weekends. The judge rejected this recommendation, holding that awarding the father sole custody would put the children at risk. The court faulted the assessor for not investigating the family environment more fully. In particular, the court noted that the assessor had not even inquired about the wife's allegation that the husband had killed the family's small pet dog in her presence by throwing it against a wall and striking its head with a hammer, an incident that the court found to be "important when details were brought out in evidence."

While the court ultimately did not rely on the assessments in either of these cases, the fact that they were made at all, and by professionals affiliated with court services, is of deep concern. In general, judges place significant weight on assessment reports. Further, more cases are settled on the basis of the recommendations of assessors than are litigated, with many women lacking the emotional or financial resources to challenge the recommendations in court. Many abused women facing a recommendation from an assessor that the father receive custody, joint custody, or extensive unsupervised access may feel obliged to settle the case on that basis, even if they feel concerned that this may endanger the safety of their children or themselves.

Assessors dealing with cases where spousal abuse is a factor require an understanding of the dynamics of these cases. Many abusive husbands are highly manipulative and present very well, while victims of domestic violence may not fare well in an assessment if the assessor does not appreciate their situation. Abusive men may be able to convince unsophisticated assessors into believing that there was no violence at all, or if it occurred that it was mutual or the fault of their partner, or had no effect on the children. If an assessor lacks the necessary knowledge and experience in dealing with cases where spousal abuse may be an issue, the opinion of the assessor should be disregarded or at very least heavily discounted by the court (e.g., *Haider v. Malach*, 1999). Counsel and courts must ensure that assessors in these cases are unbiased, and have

the requisite training and experience, and that assessments are conducted in a competent fashion.

It is important that the education and training of assessors go beyond a basic or introductory exposure to issues of domestic violence. As
U.S. legal scholar Clare Dalton notes, "One problem with the generic
training sessions in domestic violence that have become a staple of the
family court system is that they tend to reinforce somewhat stereotyped
notions of what it means to be a batterer or a victim" (1999). The result
of this simplistic portrayal of abuse is, however, that "much abuse goes
undetected" because "the reality of abuse is more complex and variable"
than the basic training sessions acknowledge. Assessors with a rudimen-
tary understanding of wife abuse may actually pose a greater danger to
abused women and their children than those with no training, as their
recommendations may appear to be infused with a sophistication about
the issues that make them more difficult to challenge.

PROBLEMATIC ACCESS ORDERS

The most significant cause for concern to emerge from our review of
these 42 cases was the terms on which abusive men were receiving access
to their children. Although judges generally understand that granting
custody to an abuser is not in the children's best interests, concerns
about children's safety and well being were not as apparent in judicial
decisions on access. Access can pose dangers for both children and their
mothers, particularly where it is unsupervised.

Children may be at risk of physical or emotional harm while in the
care of a parent with a history of spousal abuse, as discussed in Chapters
2 and 7. Separation may cause a man to try to control his former spouse
by manipulating the children; access may permit an abusive man to denigrate the mother to the children or to interrogate them about the
mother's conduct or relationships. There may also be a risk of physical
abuse during access visits. There have been a number of tragic cases in
Canada in which abusive men have killed their children during access
visits, feeling a loss of control or desire for revenge as a result of the separation ("Slain Toddlers," 2002; "Murder Suspect," 2002). Exchanging
the children at the beginning and end of the visit can also present an
abusive man with an opportunity to abuse the woman, verbally as well
as physically. Even ensuring that the changeover occurs in the presence
of third parties or in public places does not assure women's safety.
Women have been assaulted and even killed during access exchanges in
public places (Dalton, 1999).

Despite the dangers unsupervised access poses, courts awarded unsupervised access to men who abused their wives in most of the cases in our study (18 of 31). Supervised access was ordered in 6 cases, but generally this was to allow a father to reestablish a relationship with the children where the relationship had lapsed or where the children were fearful of their father, rather than because of concern over the impact of the father's behavior on the children during the access time. Access was denied in 7 cases, usually where the mother had been subjected to extreme levels of physical violence, where the children had also been exposed to the risk of serious harm, or where there was clear evidence that the children had been traumatized by exposure to spousal violence. For example, access was denied in D.(C.L.) v. D.(B.E.) (1999), where the three children were found to be exhibiting signs of "post traumatic distress" and would sometimes enter into a "dissociative, trance-like state at the mention of the father's name." Access was also ultimately denied in A.(P.) v. A.(F.) (1997), where the wife had been subjected to prolonged physical, sexual, and emotional abuse. The father had also sexually abused the two daughters, ages 6 and 9 at the time of trial, and had physically abused the two sons by beating them with canes and electrical cords. Once when one of the sons attempted to protect the mother, the father forced the child's head into the toilet and flushed. Even on these facts, the court had initially awarded supervised access, but the children refused to participate because they were fearful of their father and concerned about their mother's safety.

Generally, however, men who abused their female partners were granted access awards that look much like the standard access order courts make in nonviolence cases—access on alternate weekends, perhaps with an additional visit 1 day during the week. As reviewed in detail in Chapter 7, while unsupervised access may be appropriate in some cases despite a finding of spousal abuse, in some of the cases in our sample the decision to allow unsupervised access was troubling because it seemed to place the child or the mother at risk.

One example of this type of case is L.(C.R.) v. L.(R.F.) (1998), in which unsupervised access was awarded to a man who had not only abused his wife and children during the marriage but had also been abusive in three other intimate relationships, one of which had taken place after separation. Although the husband admitted there had been physical altercations in all four relationships, he denied any responsibility for the violence, attributing it instead to emotional problems from which he claimed all four women suffered. Two different assessors, both of whom expressed serious concern about the father's violence, his refusal to accept responsibility for his violence, and his lack of parenting ability, had prepared assessments. Both recommended that the father have limited access (one recommended that access be supervised) and no overnight visits. One report specifically mentioned that because the father took out his frustrations through violence, there was a real risk that he would lash out and hurt the children during access. Despite these assessments, the judge ordered unsupervised weekend access, observing that the children had a positive relationship with their father and that they benefited from their contact with him. The court also held that "Contact with each parent is valuable, and the only circumstance in which contact with either parent can be limited is where the contact is shown to conflict with the best interests of the child."

In another case, *C.(A.C.) v. G.(I.C.)* (1999), the court awarded a father unsupervised overnight access to his 3-year-old daughter, notwithstanding its finding that there was "overwhelming evidence" that the father had been physically and emotionally abusive to the mother, that the father was "jealous and possessive" of her, that he exercised a "reign of tyranny" over her, and that, as a result of this abusive behavior, he had a "weakened capacity to act as an appropriate role model and custodial parent." The abuse against the mother included slapping and kicking her and, on one occasion, striking her in the head with such force that she suffered permanent hearing loss. The father had been involved in at least one other abusive relationship and had three unrelated convictions for assault and aggravated assault. Although the father admitted to using violence against the mother and against his previous partner, he testified that the women had been the aggressors and that "[e]very woman I get involved with wants to beat me up." The father also admitted to having tried to "train" the mother and to telling her "I will hunt you down and kill you" if she tried to remove the child from his custody. The judge described the father's testimony in court as "aggressive and self-serving" and as amounting to a "continuation of his abuse" of the mother. When asked about his plan for caring for his 3-year-old daughter if he succeeded in his claim for custody, he responded by saying simply that the child was his "best friend."

In both of these cases, the orders for unsupervised access are troubling because there appears to be a high likelihood that access would expose the children to physical or emotional harm. Both cases illustrate a serious concern raised by Linda Neilson et al. (2001) in a comprehensive study of custody and access cases in New Brunswick, that women leaving abusive relationships are not encouraged to seek limitations on their spouse's access. Neilson found that lawyers routinely advise their clients that, in the absence of strong evidence of serious physical abuse of a child, abusive men will get unsupervised access, and that lawyers discourage mothers from seeking to deny access or requesting supervision. Advice of this sort may account for why the mother in *L.(C.R.)* agreed to unsupervised weekend access and why the mother in *C.(A.C.)* did not request supervised access at all. Neilson also reported that many of the women were concerned about the safety of access arrangements, with some being "terrified" that their children would not return home from access visits safely. An Australian study monitoring 3 years of practice (1996–1999) also found that the majority of women leaving abusive relationships agreed to arrangements or were subject to access orders on terms that did not allow them to feel that they and their children were safe (Rhoades et al., 2000). Most of the women had wanted supervised access and "no overnight stays with the father."

Studies from Canada and other jurisdictions found that access orders made in cases of domestic violence are a source of serious concern. For example, Neilson et al. (2001) found that judges seldom deny access to abusive men or order supervised access, leading her to observe that "evidence of partner abuse is considered important when making decisions about which parent should have primary care of the children, but is considered unimportant in access or contact disputes." She and her colleagues also concluded that "while in theory, the sole consideration in custody and access determinations is the best interests of the child," in reality "contact has first priority, best interests of the child second priority in access determinations." An Australian study reported a similar presumption that access should occur, particularly in terms of access orders made at the interim stage, even in abusive relationships (Rhoades et al., 2000). In the United States, the Family Violence Project of the National Council of Juvenile and Family Court Judges (1995) also found that judges "almost never deny abusive parents access to their children" and that "few judges propose protective limitations on visitation . . . and even fewer limit access to supervised visitation."

These studies support our conclusion that access orders remain a source of danger for abused women and their children, as courts often order unsupervised access where the more prudent course would be to suspend access temporarily or to order supervision. In part, the courts' reluctance to order supervised access may be explained by the shortage of supervised access facilities, as well as the view that supervised access distorts the parent–child interaction. More fundamentally, however, the tendency to grant access, and to do so on an unsupervised basis, stems from the assumption—which has become gospel in family law—that contact with both parents is virtually always in the children's best interests. This view is discussed in detail in Chapter 7. Judges are not the only players in the justice system influenced by the belief in the importance of access. Many assessors, mediators, and lawyers also subscribe to this belief, with the result (as noted above) that lawyers rarely advise clients to seek to suspend or limit contact, even in cases of wife abuse. In giving this advice, lawyers may also be affected by the "friendly parent" presumption, reflected in subsection 16(10) of Canada's *Divorce Act,* which provides that a child should "have as much contact" with each parent as is "consistent with the best interests of the child," and in dealing with custody, "the court shall take into consideration the willingness" of each parent "to facilitate such contact." As Clare Dalton (1999) puts it:

> Ironically, within the friendly parent framework, a mother's proper concern about her abusive partner's fitness to parent will negatively affect her chance to win custody, not his. At the same time, the abuser's willingness to share the children, which assures his ongoing access to his partner and allows him to continue to manipulate and intimidate her, will, within the same framework, make him appear the more attractive candidate for custody.

The confluence of these factors—the prevailing view of the importance of access for children's development, the friendly parent rule, and the implicit assumption that fathers have the right to see their children— means that access is the norm, even in cases in which the court accepts that there is a significant history of wife abuse. It also means that courts tend to award access based on a "standard" pattern developed in cases where violence was not an issue, unless they have compelling evidence not to do so. In making these awards, however, courts can be placing women and children at risk, sometimes with deadly consequences.

The finding that access is a problem for abused women and their children across jurisdictions indicates that the prevailing approach to access needs to be rethought. In small measure, this may already be taking place. Recent studies show that "the best predictors of children's well-being after separation and divorce, in *high conflict families,* are the psychological well-being of the primary caregiver and the children's freedom from continued exposure to abuse" (Neilson et al., 2001). In high-conflict families, positive outcomes for children are *not* associated with more frequent contact with noncustodial parents, and access can be a major source of stress for children. These studies clearly suggest that the justice system should develop a very different approach to access in high conflict and abuse cases.

SUMMARY AND CONCLUSIONS

Although some judges are clearly less sensitive to the issue than others, leading Canadian decisions now recognize the importance of spousal abuse as a factor in custody decisions. Many judges appreciate the need for differentiated responses depending on the nature of the abuse, the effects of that abuse on the children, the prognosis for the future, as well as the risk of immediate harm. It is, however, also clear that too often judges, lawyers, mediators, assessors, police, and other professionals fail to adequately recognize and deal with spousal abuse issues, and that too often women and children are endangered as a result. Survivors of abuse can be pressured by circumstances, a lack of resources, and a lack of effective advocacy into accepting resolutions that leave them and their children vulnerable to further abuse. Judges, lawyers, and mediators all have a role in helping them to resist these pressures.

Our study provides additional evidence to support a reassessment of the approach to the issue of postseparation access. At the most fundamental level, there is a need to think carefully about the purported benefits of access, and creatively about what maintaining contact entails. All of the key players in the justice system—judges, lawyers, assessors, mediators, and governments—need to engage in this rethinking process. Law reform should also be part of the rethinking process. In our view, all Canadian jurisdictions should enact statutes that specifically acknowledge the significance of domestic violence for child-related proceedings. Canadian legislation should be modeled on that of England, Australia, New Zealand, and other jurisdictions. Violence should not be just another "best interests" factor that judges may take into account. Rather, courts should be required to be satisfied that any parenting arrangements do not pose a significant risk to the safety of a child or parent. The enactment of such legislation would clarify the law as well as facilitate the education of lawyers, judges, other professionals, victims, and members of the public.

Statutory reform is a relatively small part of a process of change needed to protect survivors of domestic violence and their children. Enforcement issues are critical to ensure that the remedies afforded to victims of abuse, such as restraining orders, are effective. There is also a need for appropriate support services for survivors of domestic violence, including counseling for women and children, programs for abusive spouses, and facilities to supervise access. There is also a need for survivors to have adequate access to legal aid in family law cases. These cases place great demands on the lawyers who are representing victims, and they require adequate time to deal with the challenging and contentious issues they raise.

The results of our study suggest that all justice system professionals working with divorcing couples, including lawyers, judges, police, assessors, and mediators, need the knowledge and training to deal effectively with situations where spousal abuse is at issue, and in particular should be aware of the risks faced by victims of abuse and their children. These professionals must appreciate that spousal abuse covers a broad range of conduct. Given the wide range of abusive spousal conduct and the large proportion of separations and divorces that involve at least one incident of spousal abuse, the justice system and the professionals who work in it need to develop differentiated responses that take account of the specific situation of abuse and its effect on the particular parents and children involved.

NOTES

1. The term "access" is used in Canada. In the United States this is referred to as "visitation," while in the United Kingdom the term "contact" is used. These are all legal terms for a similar concept, the specification by a court or agreement of the frequency and circumstances in which the noncustodial parent will have care or visitation with the children of the relationship.

REFERENCES

Bala, N. (1999). A report from Canada's 'gender war zone': Reforming the child related provisions of the Divorce Act. *Canadian Journal of Family Law, 16,* 163–227.

Bala, N., Bertrand, L., Paetsch, J., Knoppers, B., Hornick, J., Noel, J.-F., Boudreau, L., & Miklas, S. (1998). *Spousal violence in custody and access disputes: Recommendations for reform.* Ottawa, Canada: Status of Women Canada.

Canadian Panel on Violence Against Women. (1993). *Changing the Landscape: Ending Violence, Achieving Equality.* Ottawa, Canada: Minister of Supply and Services Canada.

Dalton, C. (1999). *When paradigms collide: Protecting battered parents and their children in the Family Court System,* 37 Fam. & Conciliation Courts Rev. 273.

Family Violence Project of the National Council of Juvenile and Family Court Judges. (1995). *Family Violence in Child Custody Statutes: An Analysis of State Codes and Legal Practice.* 29, F.L.Q. 197.

Lemon, N. (2001). Statutes creating rebuttable presumptions against custody to batterers: How effective are they? *William Mitchell Law Review, 28,* 601.

Murder suspect accused wife of affair. (2002, March 18). *National Post,* p. A7.

Neilson, L. C., Baird, B., Charnley, A., Davis, C., Gallagher, T., Gavin, S., Guravich, M., Richardson, C. J., & McAllen, S. (2001). *Spousal abuse, children and the legal system.* Final report for Canadian Bar Association, Law for the Futures Fund, University of New Brunswick.

Rhoades, H., Graycar, R., & Harrison, M. (2000). The Family Law Reform Act 1995: The First Three Years. *Australian Family Lawyer, 15,* 76–77 and 79–80.

Shaffer, M. (in press). The impact of wife abuse on child custody and access determinations. *Canadian Family Law Quarterly.*

Slain toddler's father to face first-degree murder charge. (2002, March 18). *National Post*, p. A7.

Statistics Canada (2001). *Family Violence in Canada: A Statistical Profile* (p. 26). Ottawa, Canada: Canadian Centre for Justice Statistics.

FAMILY LAW CASES CITED

A.(P.) v. A.(F.) [1997] B.C.J. No. 1566 (B.C.S.C.) (QL).

C.(A.C.) v. G.(I.C.) [1999] B.C.J. No. 963 (B.C. Prov. Ct.) (QL).

Cadeau v. Martell [1998] N.S.J. No. 159 (N.S. Fam. Ct.) (QL).

D.(C.L.) v. D.(B.E.) [1999] N.B.J. No. 436 (B.B.Q.B.) (QL.).

Haider v. Malach [1999] S.J. 315 (Sask. C.A.) (QL).

L.(C.R.) v. L. (R.F.) [1998] S.J. No. 20 (Sask. Q.B.) (QL).

M.(G.E.) v. M.(C.) [1999] M.J. No. 273 (Man. Q.B.) (QL).

Mbaruk v. Mbaruk [1997] B.C.J. No. 215 (B.C.S.C.) (QL.).

Peterson v. Peterson [1998] N.S.J. No. 255 (N.S.Co.Ct) (QL.).

V.(L.). v. B(T.). [2000] N.J. No. 63 (U.F.Ct.) (QL).

12

The Role of Family Courts in Domestic Violence

The U.S. Experience

BILLIE LEE DUNFORD-JACKSON

Thirty years ago, little was known and even less written about domestic violence. Problems within a family were considered to be just that—private matters that happened behind closed doors. Any public response was considered to be interference and, thus, unseemly. Largely paralleling the evidence provided in Chapter 11 about Canada, over the past 15 years in the United States advocates for victims of domestic violence have become relatively successful in convincing judges, police, prosecutors, and other systems players that assaultive behavior against a family member is every bit as criminal as against a stranger and should be treated no less severely. During this era, the general attitude has been that perpetrators who abuse their intimate partners generally do not abuse the children as well and that, as long as the children themselves are not the direct target of the violence, they probably are not sustaining harm.

Within the past few years, however, experts on domestic violence and child development have recognized the error of these assumptions (Edleson, 2000). Partner abuse and child abuse are often two aspects of a multifaceted problem within a family; and even when direct child abuse is not a factor, children are put at increased risk of various kinds of harm by living in a home where violence occurs, as discussed in Chapter 2. Regardless of a child's individual experience, the risks of physical, behavioral, and emotional injury are substantially higher than for children who do not suffer exposure to domestic violence.

As public discourse about the potential impact of violence on children has become more widespread and sophisticated, state legislatures have responded by enacting various types of laws, some civil and some criminal, intended to protect children in homes where domestic violence has occurred, and to increase abuser accountability. Each of these approaches is well-intentioned and has the potential to help. But each brings with it the potential as well for unintended and undesirable consequences.

LEGISLATIVE APPROACHES

Custody Factors

For years, most states have included a list of factors for judges to weigh in determining how to structure custody or access and visitation decisions, as part of their child custody laws. Such factors generally include a consideration of which parent:

- Can provide greater stability for the children.
- Is more likely to put the needs of the children first.
- Has been the primary caretaker.
- Is more likely to foster a healthy relationship and frequent contacts between the children and the other parent (the so-called friendly parent provision).

One legislative response to the growing awareness of the impact of domestic violence on children, an approach adopted by almost all states at this point, is to include whether either parent has engaged in domestic violence. Although considering this factor certainly is appropriate in determining the best interests of the children, the problem is that the states generally do not address what weight the courts should accord a finding of domestic violence. For example, the judge may find that the father has a higher income and is in a better position than is the mother to maintain the family home and keep the children in the same schools and activities, enjoying the same standard of living as before the dissolution; but that, on the other hand, he has been the perpetrator of violence against the mother. Few of the state statutes offer the courts guidance in balancing these factors against one another in cases such as this.

The interplay of the domestic violence factor with the "friendly parent" factor seems to give the courts the most difficulty. The typical statute tells them to look with favor on the parent more likely to cooperate with the other in decision making concerning the children and in making them accessible for visitation. Where there has been domestic violence, the perpetrator is likely to favor custody arrangements that offer the parents the fewest restrictions on access to the children and to each other. By contrast, the victim parent will naturally favor any arrangement that calls for the least possible contact between the two adults and that best protects the children from the opportunity for the abuser to manipulate or harm them further. Given the demands of their dockets and the complicated nature of these cases, it is often difficult for courts, particularly without considerable training and experience in domestic violence, to sort all of this out. The risk is that judges may see the abuser's manipulative behavior as cooperation and the victim's protective behavior as hostility.[1]

Rebuttable Presumption against Custody for an Abuser

Roughly 40% of the states have gone a step further and have enacted a rebuttable presumption that it is not in the best interest of children to be placed in the joint or sole custody of a parent who has committed domestic violence. In these states, once the court makes a finding that domestic violence has occurred, the burden shifts to the abusing parent to prove to the court that it is in fact in the children's best interest for the abuser to have a custodial role.

The first states to pass rebuttable presumption statutes tended to offer the courts little guidance as to what it takes to reach a finding of domestic violence sufficient to trigger the presumption, or how the presumption might be rebutted. The evidence presented to courts in domestic violence cases often appears contradictory. The only witnesses may be the parties. Both may be injured, the victim from the perpetrator's assault and the perpetrator from the victim's self-defensive actions. They may each give testimony blaming the other. Or the victim, recognizing on the part of the perpetrator behavior that historically has preceded an assault, may strike first to avoid yet another beating. Without guidance from the statute as to the burden of proof necessary to trigger the presumption or how it might be rebutted, the courts in such cases are at risk of mistaking victims for perpetrators; and victims are at risk of losing custody of their children to perpetrators. Additionally, these early statutes fostered the perception that parents motivated by a desire to gain an edge in custody battles could easily abuse the rebuttable presumption provisions by making false allegations of domestic violence.

The more recent rebuttable presumption statutes tend to be more specific about what level of domestic violence must occur to trigger the effects of the statute. Some of these require a history of domestic violence or a single act that results in severe physical injury. Some require conviction of a crime of domestic violence. While these versions may reduce the likelihood that the inappropriate parent will lose custody of the children or that false allegations will succeed, at the same time they offer no relief in cases where the abusive parent uses tactics of power and control that may be equally harmful but that do not meet the statutory requirement to trigger the presumption. And rebuttable presumption statutes in general, regardless of how justifiable and specific they are, appear to create a backlash effect among the segment of the population who do not understand the dynamics of domestic violence and assert that men in general are treated unfairly in custody and visitation decisions.[2]

Separate Crime of Committing Domestic Violence in the Presence of a Child

A few states have enacted one form or another of a statute creating a separate crime of committing domestic violence in the presence of a child. Utah (§76-5-109.1) provides that a person who commits domestic violence in the presence of a child is guilty of child abuse, which may be a misdemeanor or a felony, depending upon the severity and frequency of the behavior. Oregon (§163.160) provides that domestic violence elevates from a Class A misdemeanor to a Class C felony when committed in the presence of a child. In Delaware, when a person commits an act of violence against a victim in the presence of a child of either the perpetrator or the victim (§1102), the perpetrator is guilty of the Class A misdemeanor of endangering the welfare of a child. Similarly, under Georgia law (§16-5-70), a person commits the second degree misdemeanor of cruelty to children by committing an act of domestic violence while knowing that a child is present or sees or hears the act.

Proponents advocate such laws as a means of emphasizing that domestic violence is harmful to children, and that society needs to change historic norms and attitudes that tolerate and foster such behavior. Their hope is to put the needs of these children on the radar screen of first responders, and to afford them access to resources that might be available through crime victim compensation funds. Some see these statutes as a way of getting the child protection system involved for assessment and intervention services, although (as will be discussed more fully later) that result can bring with it significant adverse consequences as well (Jaffe, Crooks, & Wolfe, 2003).

To the extent that statutes creating separate crimes for domestic violence in the presence of children achieve the hopes of their proponents, they do so at risk of severe negative repercussions. For example, in jurisdictions with such statutes, children are more likely drawn into the criminal process, with the potential for many and varied adverse consequences for them and their families. They face becoming court witnesses in the context of a system ill prepared to make accommodations for their stage of development and traumatic experience (Jaffe et al., 2003). They may suffer potential negative impact from being called to testify against one of their parents. Victims who, for whatever safety reasons, have chosen not to participate in the prosecution of their abusers may see their children called to testify against those very abusers, or may experience pressure to testify against their abusers, at whatever increased peril to themselves and their children (CEVS, 2003).

If the past is any indicator of the future, there is a strong potential for victims of domestic violence to become entangled in the web of these new crimes. For example, victims may be (1) charged as accessories to the crime of committing domestic violence in a child's presence, (2) charged with failing to protect children by not removing them from the arena of conflict, or (3) charged with committing acts of domestic violence in the presence of children by acting to defend themselves and their children from batterers' assaults (Dunford-Jackson, 1998). As happened with proarrest policies in cases of domestic violence, they may suffer contempt of court charges for unwillingness to testify and charges of perjury for changing their stories. Even worse, they may be swept up by these laws and charged as abusers themselves, as evidenced by the difficulties police experience in identifying primary aggressors (Jaffe et al., 2003).

As with any new body of legislation, enacting these statutes is one thing, while implementing them is another. Particularly in the case of crimes involving families, where effective implementation depends heavily on a wide variety of systems players—police, prosecutors, and the judiciary—being appropriately resourced and trained, the risk is that enactment of these statutes will outstrip the capacity of communities to enforce them appropriately and effectively. The result is that the system may revictimize the very victims the laws are designed to protect. These complications may create a chilling effect on the willingness of victims and children to disclose violence and seek help (Jaffe et al., 2003).

Finally, these new laws have the potential to increase the disproportionate representation of people of color in the penal system. Regrettably, an accused person from the nondominant culture is more likely to be arrested; once arrested, is more likely to be prosecuted; once prosecuted, is more likely to be convicted; and once convicted, is more likely to be punished more severely. This last factor has especially grave implications in view of a second type of criminal statute that many states have recently enacted, namely, the one that provides for increased penalties when acts of domestic violence take place where children are aware they are occurring (CEVS, 2003).

Increased Penalties for Acts of Domestic Violence Committed in the Presence of a Child

Roughly one-third of the states have opted to increase the penalty usually given for domestic violence if it occurs where a child hears, sees, or is aware of it, rather than create a separate crime. Some of the same arguments advanced for the creation of separate crimes apply in this instance: enhancing penalties is likely to bring home to still unaware policymakers and others the potential of harm to children exposed to domestic violence. At the state level, it is possible that legislative or administrative changes to laws or regulations governing crime victim funding could bring these children into the class of victims eligible for these funds, identifying them as a result of the same evidence used to prove the crime. When police document the presence of children at the scene, they may be more likely to report to child protective services, thereby triggering services for these children.

Certainly, enhanced penalties serve the goal of holding abusers accountable for the harm they cause the children exposed to their violence; and certainly they provide a sanction for abusers who are not biologically related to the children and so are unlikely to be reachable in any other way that is meaningful to them (CEVS, 2003). On the other hand, it still happens with disturbing frequency that victims of domestic violence are themselves charged with domestic violence crimes when they seek to defend themselves or protect their children. Heightened penalties apply to anyone convicted of the charge, whether the abuser or the inappropriately charged victim. Enhanced penalties may increase the danger that the perpetrator poses to the victim. Because he faces additional criminal penalties as a result of committing acts of violence in front of the children, he may be more likely to pressure the victim to drop the case and may increase the level of threats and violence to keep her from testifying. Or, he may threaten the children to prevent them from testifying. Especially if he is acquitted, his retribution against victim and children may be more severe (CEVS, 2003).

Both criminalization and increased penalties have the potential to hurt the justice system itself. They impose greater costs on the system by involving greater numbers of offenders for longer periods of time without producing appreciable benefits for children. In fact, while some children may feel vindicated by having a hand in holding the abusers of their parents accountable, others may feel guilty and estranged from either or both parents. The resources consumed by these new crimes may divert much-needed funds from programs and initiatives that could provide greater benefits to children and their nonabusive parents. More prosecutions, more convictions, longer sentences, more children in foster care, the need for more personnel in the police and child protection agencies that will feel this impact, the risk of professional burnout, and the need for constant recruitment and training of replacements—all of these are foreseeable outcomes from the approach of creating a new domestic violence crime or making current penalty structures more severe (CEVS, 2003).

Finally, the new criminal approaches, whether criminalization or increased penalties, compound the problem of the mixed message received by families caught in the nightmare of domestic violence. These families are frequently involved with multiple courts, handling various causes of action arising from the same incidents. Creating a separate crime for domestic violence committed in the presence of a child, or "enhancing" criminal penalties for such acts, sends a loud, clear signal in criminal court that domestic violence in the presence of children is so harmful to them that it is being singled out for special attention and treatment. At the same time that an abuser is facing these charges in criminal court, the family may be in dependency court, again because the potential for harm to the children is so great that the system feels called upon to intervene in their behalf and perhaps even to remove them from their home. And while all of this is going on, this same family may be in family court, where the victim hears that contact with their other parent, the abuser, is so important to the children that she faces contempt of court and even loss of custody to that very abuser if she fails to make them available for visitation. Or, she may face joint custody and joint decision making with the same abuser who is deemed in the other court settings to be a dire threat to her and the children. Or, she may be accused of alienating the children from him because they are reluctant to spend time with him. In fact, it is not uncommon for the victim to be subject at the same time to two inconsistent orders, one from dependency court prohibiting her from permitting contact between the batterer and the children on pain of being found to have failed to protect them, and one from family court requiring her to make the children available for visitation with the abuser. Such inconsistencies among the philosophies underlying various court proceedings may put both nonabusing parents and their children at even greater risk (CEVS, 2003).

Statutes Affecting Child Protection Proceedings

A number of statutory developments that directly impact child dependency courts and proceedings parallel the activity in the criminal realm in response to concerns about children exposed to domestic violence. There are two main types of these statutes: (1) those that make a wide variety of systems players mandatory reporters of child abuse and require the reporting to child protective services of any children exposed to domestic violence; and (2) those that broaden the statutory definition of child abuse to include exposing a child to domestic violence. As with the other statutes discussed in this chapter, these are intended to protect children from harm, and they arise from the premise that exposure to violence is equally as abusive as physical or sexual abuse. They give the public a clear message that domestic violence is unacceptable and that children are its secondary victims. They establish the unacceptability of domestic violence as a social norm and may cause parents to take greater care to avoid exposing their children to violent behavior. They may trigger such immediate services for children in violent homes as counseling, support, and protection (Jaffe et al., 2003).

However well intentioned these statutory developments, they have on occasion had devastating consequences. For example, Florida enacted a law naming judges as mandatory reporters of child abuse. At the same time, the state's child protective services agency was interpreting the Florida child abuse statute to include exposing children to domestic violence. As a result, when victims of domestic violence gave information on applications for protection orders that indicated children had been in the house during acts of violence, the courts reported these children to the child protection agency. Many of these children were at least temporarily removed from their homes and put into foster care. Victims soon stopped seeking relief from the courts for themselves and their children. The agency has since changed its interpretation of the child abuse statute.

Minnesota similarly passed a statute mandating the reporting of all children exposed to domestic violence. Within a short time, reported cases overwhelmed the child protection system, to the extent that the best the agency could do was try to assess each case. This effort to assess

the flood of cases consumed all resources, so that services became unavailable even for children indicated by the assessment process to have
the direst need. Six months later, the state legislature rescinded the statute.

An even stronger argument against either of these two legislative
approaches is the inaccuracy of the assumption underpinning these laws:
that children exposed to domestic violence require the same level of
community support as children who are the direct victims of physical
and sexual abuse. On the contrary, as discussed in Chapter 2, research
reveals that not all children so exposed experience significant emotional
and behavioral problems. While some may suffer significant short- or
long-term adjustment problems, others have normal development, apparently because they are able to benefit from various resources and protective factors in their lives (Edleson, 2000). Any legislation that widens
the net to catch all children who witness domestic violence fails to take
into account their variability in response and therefore brings into the
system many children who do not need to be there. The result puts additional stressors on the already overburdened system that it may not be
able to bear, as in the Minnesota experience. It may also revictimize and
disempower abused mothers.

In fact, as previously discussed in Chapter 2, the Nicholson case, recently decided in the Eastern District of New York, provides a textbook
example of how the presumption that witnessing abuse harms all children who witness it—the presumption underlying the enactment of all of
the legislation described in this chapter—can lead to indefensible results
(Stark, 2002). Nicholson was a class action suit against the Administration for Children Services and the City of New York on behalf of women
whose children were removed from their custody and placed in foster
care because these mothers had failed to protect the children by allowing
them to be exposed to domestic violence (in the agency's language, these
women were "engaging in domestic violence" in the presence of the children). At least one of the named plaintiffs in the lawsuit had separated
herself and her children from her abuser at the same time she sought assistance from the system, so that whatever danger the children had suffered no longer existed by the time the state became involved. Neverthe-
less, in the agency's estimation this mother had failed to protect her
children; therefore, they were taken into foster care. Fortunately, the
Nicholson court found these actions by the New York child protection
agency inappropriate, issued an opinion requiring the agency to revamp
its procedures, and put in place guidelines for the agency to obtain the
guidance of experts in the field to assist with the revamping process. The
court based part of its opinion in this case on *Effective Interventions in*

Domestic Violence and Child Maltreatment Cases: Guidelines for Policy and Practice (the Greenbook), published by the National Council of Juvenile and Family Court Judges in 1999. The Greenbook acknowledges the high overlap between domestic violence and child maltreatment and the resulting fact that child protective services, domestic violence service providers, and dependency courts often intervene in the same families at the same time. However, traditionally, these three systems have focused only on the aspect of the problem in which each has expertise, have failed to communicate with each other or to coordinate their services and interventions, and have often worked at cross-purposes with each other, to the detriment of the families they attempt to serve. The Greenbook treats the nonviolent members of the family as a unit with common interests and offers recommendations, directed at each of these three systems, for improving their interventions and coordinating their efforts.

SUMMARY AND CONCLUSIONS

The Greenbook provides testimony that not all system interventions are bad. Certainly domestic violence is a societal plague that needs to end. Certainly we, as a society, should take steps to help families afflicted by this plague. Certainly, no matter how resilient an individual child may be, exposure to domestic violence is not helpful. The catch is figuring out how to put in place interventions that help individual victims and children. A major key to formulating beneficial interventions seems to lie in avoiding the one-size-fits-all approach that stems from the false assumption that exposure to domestic violence constitutes child abuse per se. Avoiding iron-clad rules is the approach encouraged by the Greenbook, whether for policy development or for legislation. Some promising statutes have recently been enacted that might serve as good examples. For example, Alaska law (AK§47.10.011, 47.17.020) permits a court to find a child who has been exposed to domestic violence in need of aid for the purposes of obtaining such services as the child may need, but on the other hand allows the mandatory reporter to make an exception and not report such a child if the reporter has reasonable cause to believe the child is safe and not presently in danger of mental injury because of the exposure.

To cite another example, under Oregon law (§411.117), the Department of Social Services must (1) screen its caseload for domestic violence, (2) offer individualized case management to cases involving domestic violence, and (3) waive or modify the usual requirements that might place victims of domestic violence at risk (for example, time limits, work requirements, and participating in paternity determination and child support collection).

For still a third example, Minnesota recently enacted a law (§626.552) requiring that a welfare agency must consider the safety of both the child and the victimized parent in determining what protective action to take and what services to offer a child exposed to domestic violence and the child's family. In determining whether the child needs protective services, the agency must consider protective factors in the child's environment, such as (1) whether the child has been the direct target of physical or sexual abuse or neglect, (2) the child's age, (3) the length of time since exposure to the violence, (4) the child's relationship to the victim parent and to the perpetrator of the violence, and (5) whether steps have been taken to exclude the abuser from the child's home or the adult victim has sought protective services such as shelters or counseling, or advocacy services, legal recourse, or other remedies.

As different as these statutes are from one another, they have in common their nuanced approach to the complex problem of children exposed to domestic violence. They acknowledge that every family, every situation, every set of needs, is different. They call for individual assessment and a system response tailor-made for the needs of the particular people involved in a specific case. This appears to be the best way to make sure that our laws achieve the beneficial interventions that motivate them and avoid the unintended consequences that inevitably flow from treating all cases as if they are the same.

NOTES

1. Examples of statutes that list domestic violence as one factor among many for the court to consider, with no guidance provided as to the relative weight it should be given, include: AK §§25.24.150 and 25.20.090; CO §14-10-124; KS §60-1610; KY §403.270; NE §42-364; NJ §9:2–4; and VA §200-124.3. Examples of statutes that require the courts to give priority to the domestic violence factor include: AR §9-15-215; DC §16-911; GA §§19-9-1 and 19-9-3; and HI §571-46.

2. AL §30-3-133 and HI §571-46 are examples of early versions of the rebuttable presumption statute that provide simply that a finding of domestic violence triggers the presumption. Among the later statutes that set more specific standards and, in some cases, address how to rebut the presumption once it has been raised, are: CA Fam §3044, which provides that a finding by the court of domestic violence within the 5 years prior to the hearing raises the presumption; and that the presumption can be rebutted by a preponderance of the evidence that it is in the best interest of the child for the abuser to

have a custodial role; FL §61.13, in which evidence of a domestic violence felony of the third degree or higher triggers the presumption; and any lesser evidence of domestic violence constitutes evidence of harm to the child and also that one of the factors to be considered in its "friendly parent" provision is whether one of the parents has committed domestic violence against the other; ID §32-717B, providing that a finding by the court that one parent is a habitual perpetrator of domestic violence raises the presumption against joint custody; IA §598.41, which provides that a finding by the court that domestic violence occurred raises the presumption and also, in the friendly parent provision, that domestic violence by one parent is justification for the other not to cooperate in making the children available to the maximum extent possible; MA 209c §10, in which a finding by a preponderance of the evidence either of a pattern or of one serious event of domestic violence raises the presumption; and that the presumption is rebuttable by a preponderance of evidence that a perpetrator custodial role is in child's best interest; NV §14-09-06.2, requiring credible evidence of one serious event or a pattern of domestic violence within a relevant timeframe in order for the presumption to apply, and allowing rebuttal by clear and convincing evidence that the best interest of the child requires the perpetrator's participation as a custodial parent; and OK 43 §112.2, requiring clear and convincing evidence of ongoing domestic violence in order for the presumption to apply.

REFERENCES

The Children Exposed to Violence Subcommittee for the Greenbook Policy Advisory Committee (CEVS). (2003). *Guidlines for testing proposed policies and legislative changes regarding children exposed to domestic violence.* Unpublished.

Dunford-Jackson, B. L. (1998). Creation of new crimes/enhanced penalties for commission of domestic violence in the presence of a child. *Synergy, 3*(2).

Edelson, J. (2000). *Should childhood exposure to adult domestic violence be defined as child maltreatment under the law?* Available at *http://www.mincava. umn.edu/link.*

Jaffe, P. G., Crooks, C. V., & Wolfe, D. A. (2003). Legal and policy responses to children exposed to domestic violence: The need to evaluate intended and unintended consequences. *Clinical Child and Family Psychology Review, 6,* 205–213.

Stark, E. (2002). *The battered mother in the child protective service caseload: Developing an appropriate response.* 23 Women's Rts. L. Rep. 107.

13

The Fourth R

*Developing Healthy Relationships
through School-Based Interventions*

PETER G. JAFFE, DAVID WOLFE,
CLAIRE CROOKS, RAY HUGHES, and LINDA L. BAKER

Recent episodes of lethal violence in schools have made every parent, teacher, and student more aware of violence in schools and much more conscious of safety (Garbarino, 1999). Numerous initiatives have arisen, ranging from an attempt by the FBI to create a profile of a "school shooter" to specific inquests, such as the one following the tragedy at Columbine High School in Littleton, Colorado (Erickson, 2001). As questions of accountability and liability are raised, it is increasingly clear that school violence is being taken extremely seriously; unfortunately, there is still much confusion about how to direct efforts to address this concern.

The Columbine incident, in particular, led to a widespread feeling of "if it can happen there, it can happen anywhere." Columbine High

School is an upper-middle-class suburban school with high scholastic standards (Erickson, 2001). It is well known for the success of its athletic teams, and a large majority of its graduates go on to college. The Columbine incident mirrored previous incidents of school shootings in that, according to the Columbine Commission report (Erickson, 2001), the perpetrators were students who had been bullied at school and who were seeking to kill students and teachers that they knew. This reality that youths are more likely to experience violence at the hands of somebody they know is at the heart of the "Fourth R" concept. The Fourth R is intended to draw attention to the importance of relationships both in understanding violence and in knowing how to prevent it.

The majority of violence is inherently relational in nature; despite the myth of assault by strangers, surveys in the United States and Canada indicate that most children are victimized by people they know and trust (Wolfe & Jaffe, 2001). Furthermore, the need for providing "relationship education" in addition to the other three R's (reading, writing, 'rithmetic) has never been more pronounced. Changing the norms and climate about relationships and providing students and teachers with the skills needed to foster healthy relationships is the only viable way to shift from a crisis orientation to one of prevention in response to school violence. Unfortunately, relationships remain the neglected "R" in most school settings.

The picture of our current progress in violence prevention is not uniformly bleak. Police and shelters for abused women have encouraged schools to get involved in violence prevention and have faced resistance as to the legitimacy of this endeavor in an academic environment. The good news is that now the role of schools is no longer debated; indeed, many educators want to be leaders in the effort against violence. The bad news is that people are still looking for quick solutions; find the bad kids and suspend or expel them, and have more physical security and monitoring. Furthermore, the emphasis continues to be on extreme and stranger-perpetrated violence rather than the daily reality of bullying, harassment, and abuse in the context of peer and intimate relationships.

A comprehensive approach to violence faced by school-age children and youth must recognize that many youth are exposed to violence in their families. In an average classroom, there might be three to five children dealing with the aftermath of being abused or exposed to violence in their own home (Sudermann, Jaffe, & Schieck, 1996) (see Chapter 3 for a full discussion of the incidence of children exposed to domestic violence). In addition, discussions of harassment in the school environment have to include the fact that the perpetrator may be a peer, but may also be a trusted adult such as a parent (Wolfe & Jaffe, 2001) or teacher (Robins, 2000).

The role of peers and trusted adults in perpetrating school-based abuse has not received the same media coverage as discrete episodes of lethal violence for two reasons: (1) Day-to-day harassment by peers is not as sensational as a Columbine-type incident unless it culminates in serious injury or death; and (2) The recognition that adults working within our trusted institutions can and do violate the youths they are expected to protect is painful for educators and the public to address. Finally, although domestic violence is the most common form of violence that children witness, there is still considerable controversy as to whether school lessons should turn a spotlight onto violence in the home, as this issue tends to be cloaked in privacy and secrecy. Thus, we are currently at a crossroads regarding the role of school-based programming in preventing violence and promoting healthy relationships.

There has never been greater awareness of, and anxiety surrounding, the issue of violence. At the same time, we have never been more polarized in deciding how to respond, reactively versus proactively. In fact, this debate touches the highly politicized debate in the youth justice arena on rehabilitation and prevention versus getting tough with boot camps and stricter sanctions. Countless sources, such as the American Psychological Association Commission on Violence and Youth, recognize the potential for schools to become a leading force in providing programs to reduce and prevent violence in adolescence (American Psychological Association, 1993). However, this potential has not been fulfilled, despite unprecedented funding in the area of violence prevention. Far from being at the cutting edge of promoting healthy relationships in a proactive way, many school boards have become increasingly entrenched in reactive, security-driven approaches.

The Columbine Commission report reflects this tension between reactivity and prevention. On the one hand, the report dedicates large sections to providing guidelines for crisis response (including improving communication during a crisis, advanced planning for critical emergencies, and using police officers assigned to a school). Other recommendations are more proactive in nature and recognize that this will be an intensive, ongoing process. In particular, the report speaks to the need to encourage students to "break the code of silence" and to instigate violence prevention programs in all schools. Indeed, the universal use of metal detectors, video surveillance, and other security equipment was unequivocally rejected as a way to deter school violence. That is, while many of the recommendations center around a more effective response in critical emergencies, there is also an acceptance that tighter security alone will not prevent further heinous incidents from occurring.

This chapter discusses the role of schools in Canada and the United States in preventing violence. Although violence prevention is equally relevant from the first day of kindergarten to the end of high school, this chapter will focus on the unique opportunity during adolescence. Next, the need for a paradigmatic approach to violence prevention in schools is discussed, followed by the introduction of the Transtheoretical Model (TTM) as a potential model that could be adapted for this purpose. An adapted model, the Stage-Based School Change Model, is presented, with a description of the needs at each stage, and examples of innovative stage-based strategies are described.

THE ROLE OF SCHOOLS IN PREVENTING VIOLENCE IN ADOLESCENCE

Schools are increasingly called on to help students develop good citizenship and character, in addition to providing a foundation of academic skills. In a cosponsored U.S. Department of Justice and Department of Education document, schools are challenged to "reinforce and promote the shared values of their local communities, such as honesty, kindness, responsibility, and respect for others" (Dwyer, Osher, & Warger, 1998). There are many advantages inherent in school-based prevention programming. The universal nature of the school experience allows for repeated opportunities over time to provide a foundation of relationship skills and nonviolent conflict resolution tactics (American Psychological Association, 1993). In addition, a true health promotion approach can be used that extends beyond a prevention model, in that all children can be taught these core skills instead of only addressing those youth deemed to be "high risk." The school setting is also the crucible in which peer socialization takes place. The inevitable peer conflicts provide the chance to foster adaptive or, conversely, challenge maladaptive patterns that may have germinated in the home environment.

Although the importance of school-based relationship skills promotion and violence prevention is widely accepted, there is a significant gap between the ideal prevention model and what currently exists in most schools. The rhetoric is one of promoting healthy relationships and preventing violence before it starts, but the majority of interventions are still reactive in nature. A nationwide study of Canadian school boards divided individual boards into one of four categories (Day, Golench, MacDougall & Beals-Gonzalez, 1995):

- Level 1: "Response/Sanctions"—boards that believe that the most effective way to deter aggression is to convey the message that "consequences will follow unacceptable behavior."
- Level 2: "Expectations for Behavior"—boards that have gone be-

yond a focus on sanctions to develop a model for appropriate behavior.

- Level 3: "Identification/Prevention"—boards that incorporate procedures for the identification and reduction of student behavior problems.
- Level 4: "Community Focus"—boards that subscribe to an intervention/prevention model.

The majority of the boards (49%) were classified as subscribing to the Response/Sanction approach. In comparison, 30% of the boards were classified as having an Expectations for Behavior approach, 18% subscribed to an Intervention/Prevention model, and only 4% had a Community Focus (Day et al., 1995).

A major component identified as part of the Response/Sanctions focus is a statement concerning suspension and expulsion. Our current heavy reliance on these types of interventions is problematic for two reasons. First, the presumed deterrent effect of strict sanctions is not supported by research, and second, this approach proclaims itself to embrace the popular concept of "zero tolerance," while in actuality the original "zero tolerance" paradigm has been constricted considerably since its application to the area of violence prevention. Zero tolerance has essentially been reduced to a slogan that offers token resistance (e.g., "just say no to drugs") but provides no blueprint for meaningful behavioral and attitude change. Funds are spent on bumper stickers rather than appropriate staff training and resources to implement prevention and intervention programs. Because of its current popularity and misunderstanding, we turn briefly to a discussion of zero tolerance.

THE EVOLUTION OF THE "ZERO TOLERANCE" CONCEPT

The term "zero tolerance" evokes a get-tough sentiment that has been politically well received. This concept has been widely applied in a number of campaigns to reduce and eliminate high-risk behaviors at a societal level (e.g., antidrug campaigns, drinking and driving efforts). The application of the term in relation to violence was introduced to the Canadian public in 1993 in the final report of the Canadian Panel on Violence Against Women (Canadian Panel on Violence Against Women, 1993). According to the report, adopting a "zero tolerance policy" meant "making a firm commitment to the philosophy that no amount of violence is acceptable, and that adequate resources must be made available to eliminate violence and achieve equality" (Canadian Panel on Violence, 1993). From this definition, it is clear that "zero tolerance" was meant as an end goal, not simply as a reactive punishment-oriented stance. The concept of accountability is an inherent part of zero tolerance, but zero tolerance was also envisioned to encapsulate a proactive action strategy. The misapplication of "zero tolerance" has been highlighted by front-page stories of a grade 1 student being suspended from school for trying to kiss a girl in his class. The real meaning of zero tolerance would be having a teacher in the classroom give immediate feedback that the behavior is inappropriate and that the physical space of others needs to be respected.

The subsequent adoption of the zero tolerance language in the school systems has focused on the first part of the definition (i.e., a commitment that violence is unacceptable) while largely ignoring the second part (i.e., the commitment of resources to formulate a proactive wide-scale behavior change strategy). The ideal application of zero tolerance to violence "has to include all aspects of society, including schools, parenting, interpersonal conflict resolution, and the media and entertainment industries" (Sudermann & Jaffe, 1998). Unfortunately, this vision of accountability and mobilization on the part of all segments of society has been reduced to a policy of expulsions and sanctions, despite the lack of empirical evidence for the efficacy of such strategies as deterrents of violent behavior.

LACK OF A PARADIGMATIC APPROACH TO SCHOOL-BASED VIOLENCE PREVENTION

Recognizing the need to balance out proactive health promotion strategies and reactive consequence-based protocols is not new. Indeed, the past decade witnessed a sharp rise in the number of programs developed to foster the skills-based side of the equation. Despite the availability of these programs, widespread adoption has not been achieved. Many of these programs have been short-lived, and their success has often depended on the enthusiasm and vision of a handful of dedicated staff. In some cases, a program lasts as long as the accompanying evaluation, then fizzles after the research team withdraws from the school. Within a particular school board there may be considerable disparity in the extent to which individual schools embrace available opportunities for violence prevention. It is clear that the issue is not simply one of resources or programs. What accounts for these differences among schools, and why is it such a struggle to get violence prevention initiatives incorporated into school systems in an ongoing, self-sustaining manner? The answer lies in the lack of a paradigmatic approach to school-based violence prevention.

Previous models that outline the steps a school needs to take to develop an antiviolence strategy tend not to account for the transition between steps. The missing piece in these models is that of motivation or intention to change. Where old-school models of therapy and change see motivation as a characteristic inherent to the individual trying to change (i.e., unsuccessful progress was often attributed to client resistance or lack of motivation), newer models, such as the transtheoretical model of change (Prochaska & DiClemente, 1983), recognize that motivation itself is an appropriate target for intervention.

THE TRANSTHEORETICAL MODEL
APPLIED TO ORGANIZATIONAL CHANGE

The transtheoretical model of change (TTM) was developed to provide a framework for explaining the way that individuals make significant behavioral change, particularly in health-related behaviors (Prochaska & DiClemente, 1983). The TTM was founded on the premise that individuals move through a predictable series of five discernible stages when undertaking behavioral change: (1) precontemplation, (2) contemplation, (3) preparation, (4) action, and (5) maintenance. Each stage is different from the others in terms of an individual's "readiness" to take action. The boundary between stages is somewhat arbitrary in that it is partially based on a temporal dimension with particular cutoffs. In addition, individuals are expected to progress through the stages with intermittent regression to previous stages before progressing onwards; thus, the process is seen as somewhat repetitive in nature.

In the *precontemplation* phase, individuals are not planning to act in the foreseeable future. They may be insufficiently informed about the consequences of their behavior or deny that the behavior poses a problem. The next stage, *contemplation,* describes an individual who recognizes that he or she has a problem and intends to change within the next 6 months. In the *preparation* stage, individuals intend to take action in the immediate future and have likely already taken some significant action within the past year. *Action* is the stage in which people make specific, observable changes in their overt behavior. The final stage, *maintenance,* describes a stage where individuals are less tempted to relapse and more confident of their ability to sustain their behavioral change. Research demonstrates that matching particular change strategies to each individual stage of change increases success and decreases dropout rates across a wide range of targeted behaviors (Prochaska & Velicer, 1997).

The TTM arose as a conceptual model for charting change primarily in health-related behavior (e.g., smoking, exercise, diet). It has subsequently been expanded to include change in social problems, such as violence perpetration, through validation of the model with men involved in batterer treatment (Levesque, Gelles, & Velicer, 2000). There has also been tentative support for the model to explain the process by which women end an abusive relationship (Burke, Carlson Gielen, McDonnell, O'Campo, & Maman, 2001). The success of the TTM in explaining change in a wide range of problem domains suggests a robustness of the model that is independent of the problem under consideration.

Although the TTM was initially developed to explain change in individuals, it has been applied more recently to change within organizations (Prochaska, Prochaska, & Levesque, 2001). This application arose out of the widespread recognition of the need for an integrated theoretical framework in the area of organizational change (e.g., Van DeVen & Poole, 1995; Pfeffer, 1993). More specifically, it was assumed that most efforts at change within organizations are unsuccessful because they are attempted without recognition of the principles of change (Porras & Robertson, 1992, cited in Prochaska et al., 2001). Although the framework for organizational change includes the same stages as the original model for individual change, the specific strategies used to move between stages are somewhat different.

A SCHOOL-BASED VIOLENCE ASSESSMENT AND VIOLENCE PREVENTION MODEL

While the TTM provides a useful framework for change in general, it requires some adaptation and elaboration to fit the case of school-based violence prevention. The steps that a school must navigate to effectively target violence are outlined by Sudermann, Jaffe, and Schieck in their school-based antiviolence program (ASAP; Sudermann et al., 1996). The steps outlined by this document include (1) naming, (2) understanding, (3) programming, (4) prevention, and (5) integration. These steps can be adapted to define the concepts of the TTM by forming a hybrid of the two models, the Stage-Based School Change Model (see Table 13.1).

The application of the Stage-Based School Change Model provides two clear advantages over the current "one-size-fits-all" approach to school-based intervention. First, the model can lead to a theoretically in-

TABLE 13.1. Comparison of Stage Characteristics in the Stage-Based School Change Model and the Transtheoretical Model of Change

Stage-based school change model[a]	Transtheoretical model[b]	Generic prototype in transtheoretical model of change	Unique characteristics in school-based violence prevention
Inertia	Precontemplation	• Denial of problem • Lack of acceptance of negative consequences associated with *not* changing	• Silence (can exist at all levels of stakeholders) • Hopelessness, helplessness • Ignorance—know violence occurs, but see it as random, discrete acts by bad individuals
Naming the problem	Contemplation	• Awareness that problem exists • Realize need for change	• Articulate commitment to address violence in school community • Perception of violence broadens to concept of it as a widespread community problem • Recognize that schools play an integral role in perpetuating or addressing violence in the larger community • Aware that remedies exist and change is possible
Understanding the problem	Preparation	• Preparing to make change in immediate future	• Three components to understanding how to address violence: 1. Role of behavioral expectations and sanctions 2. Reality that most violence occurs in relationships 3. Violence as a complex, multiply determined social issue (role of family, media, peers)
Program and policy development	Action	• Phase where observable action and attempts to change are evident	• Directly linked to how violence is understood: 1. Obedience model 2. Skill-based healthy relationship promotion model for all students; appropriate services for victims and perpetrators 3. Need to influence multiple systems and intervene before problems are entrenched 4. Recognize need for differential interventions by gender, cultural groups, experience with violence, community realities

(*continued*)

TABLE 13.1. (*continued*)

Stage-based school change model	Transtheoretical model	Generic prototype in transtheoretical model of change	Unique characteristics in school-based violence prevention
Integration and accountability	Maintenance	• Relapse prevention	• Integrated policies and goals • Community collaboration among parents, community agencies, students, and school staff • Clearly articulated responsibilities at both school and system level • Evaluation of programs • Ongoing cycle of feedback and refinements • Annual report cards documenting progress and needs for improvement

*a*Adapted from Sudermann, Jaffe, and Schieck (1996).
*b*Prochaska and DiClemente (1983).

formed assessment tool to categorize schools into the different readiness-to-change stages. A second advantage of the model is that it provides clear guidelines (and empirical support) for working with resistance to change, based on two decades of research with the TTM. Application of this model, in combination with a validated assessment tool, would increase our capacity to meet schools "where they are at." By developing the flexibility to meet individual school's needs in a systematic, theoretically informed way, we could hypothesize less likelihood of overwhelming schools and inadvertently feeding their resistance to change.

THE STAGE-BASED SCHOOL CHANGE MODEL

The stages of change as applied to school-based violence prevention bear characteristics of the TTM stages used in other domains (Prochaska et al., 2001) but also have components that reflect the uniqueness of the school setting. These characteristics are outlined in Table 13.1, and a discussion of each stage is included here.

Inertia

In this phase, there is silence about violence as a problem, and stakeholders at all levels may be overwhelmed by feelings of helplessness or hopelessness. The Inertia phase is different from the standard Precontemplation phase in that the latter is defined by the lack of awareness that a problem exists. In the case of violence, we are largely past the stage where people do not recognize the existence of the problem. Another characteristic of Inertia is recognizing that violence exists but conceptualizing it as random, discrete acts on the part of individuals who are either mentally ill or bad. Schools that focus all of their resources on the detection of these "violent individuals" are characterized as being in the Inertia phase. Such schools might react swiftly and severely to transgressions but minimize their own role in promoting healthy relationships and preventing violence.

Naming the Problem

In this phase, a school's perception of violence broadens to the concept of violence as a widespread community problem rather than the acts of a few disturbed individuals. This stage would also be the point at which a given school comes to be aware that remedies exist and change is possible, and makes a commitment to address violence in the school community. Inherent to being in this stage is a recognition that schools play an integral role in perpetuating or addressing violence in the larger community. As with all phases, different segments of the school system could be at different stages at different times. One feature identified as a necessary prerequisite of schools that are ready to change is the presence of a leader (often the principal) who is committed to the process (Stephens, 1998). The critical nature of this role is emphasized by many writers. For example, "a school administrator without a safe school plan is like a pilot without a flight plan" (Elliott, Williams, & Hamburg, 1998). Without someone willing to take a leadership role, it can be hypothesized that a school would get stuck in the Inertia phase, perhaps making brief, vague attempts to move forward.

Understanding the Problem

This stage includes three types of understanding that need to be developed. First, a school needs to understand the role of behavioral expectations and sanctions in preventing violence. Second, there needs to be a recognition that most violence occurs in relationships. Third, violence must be conceptualized as a complex, multiply determined social issue, with an appreciation of the roles played by family, media, and peers. As with the conventional Preparation stage, schools in the Understanding the Problem stage collect information about different programs and attempt to determine a suitable course of action. Committees, focus groups, and teams are hallmarks of this stage, and these groups hopefully include members of the different systems (e.g., students, teachers, administrators, and parents). The multiple components of understanding serve as the foundation for this preparatory work; if a school only understands the role of sanctions in deterring behavior, then it will prepare a program focusing solely on the implementation of such sanctions.

Program and Policy Development

Similar to the Action phase, this stage is characterized by overt activity, including psychoeducational components, policy review, poster competitions, displays, newsletters, and a high degree of teacher, administrator, parent, and student involvement. By definition, the Action phase is time-limited; even though there will be ongoing effort, the intensity of the activity level characteristic of this phase cannot be maintained indefinitely. The type of actions that a school chooses to engage in during the Program and Policy Development stage stem directly from the complexity of understanding achieved in the previous stage. One way to conceptualize the two action routes is to consider the trade-off between an obedience model and a skill development model: an obedience model focuses on well-articulated policy and clear consequences for transgressions (an inherently reactive model) and, by definition, will never be successful in preventing violence; in comparison, the skill development model focuses on teaching the necessary skills and values and creating a climate that enhances the ability of all members of the school community to play a role in preventing violence. The most effective strategy incorporates the clear expectations and structure espoused by the obedience model as well as the skill-based prevention components of a responsibility model. However, for a school to pursue the more complex solutions consistent with a skill development model requires a depth of understanding about the multiple causes and relational nature of violence that is not currently found in many schools.

Integration and Accountability

Schools in this stage (i.e., the Maintenance phase) still participate in special events such as those mentioned in the Program and Policy Development phase; however, most of the activities are self-sustaining. Skill-building activities integrated into a curriculum or regular meetings of a social action club are examples of activities in this category. In comparison to schools in the Program and Policy Development phase, these schools might not appear as outwardly busy in their pursuit of violence prevention, as many of the activities are seamlessly integrated into the everyday routine of the school. In addition to integration of programs, there is integration between systems (e.g., parents, teachers, school boards) and policies (i.e., not a separate sexual harassment policy and a separate bullying policy). Inherent to the accountability part of this stage is the notion that success in this area has to be measured and it has to matter. Schools at this stage have a strong commitment to ongoing surveillance and reassessment of their status in respect to violence prevention. Annual report cards document progress and needs for improvement (comparable to standardized testing in core academic areas) and provide a mechanism for this accountability. Finally, these schools provide a supportive role for schools that are earlier in the change process.

STAGE-SPECIFIC INTERVENTIONS

The remainder of this chapter is devoted to the types of interventions required at each step of the Stage-Based School Change Model. Examples of innovative strategies currently used in the Thames Valley District School Board (London and Middlesex, Elgin, and Oxford counties) in Ontario, Canada, are used for purpose of illustration (visit *www.tvdsb.on.ca.* for more information).

Moving from Inertia to Naming the Problem

The processes required of a school in the Inertia stage include dramatic relief, self-reevaluation, and thinking about commitment. Dramatic relief is described as the process wherein emotional arousal (such as fear about failure to change or excitement about possibility of change) is targeted to increase motivation (Prochaska et al., 2001). It is essentially the process of helping a school see that they cannot afford not to change. The Thames Valley District School Board uses a variety of performing art-based activities to evoke these emotions. Students perform plays written by students and teachers at various schools to challenge people to think about violence. Following the presentations, university students, trained as facilitators, lead discussions in small groups. Another activity used is the "Love That Kills" video (National Film Board of Canada, 1999) and accompanying discussion. This video is based on the true story of a young woman who was in an abusive relationship and was eventually murdered by her boyfriend. Both the drama presentations and the video tend to stimulate emotional reactions in students and staff, and in this capacity they help to generate momentum among a group of people regarding the need to change. It is unrealistic, however, to expect lasting behavior change on the basis of seeing one video or theater presentation.

Understanding the Problem

The core need of the Understanding the Problem stage is to shift people's thinking about violence away from an emphasis on violent individuals who must be punished to a complex relationship-based social problem with numerous contributors and opportunities for intervention. One way to approach this phase is to present people who are further along the readiness-to-act spectrum with opportunities to think about plans and share ideas with others. Approximately 100 high school students in the Thames Valley District School Board had an opportunity to engage in these processes as part of a major international conference in London, Ontario, during the summer of 2001. The conference attracted over 950 delegates, and 170 individuals presented from 19 countries. Concurrent with this conference, a special initiative for grade 11 students was organized to enable students to meet and discuss domestic and dating violence as well as to develop a plan for violence prevention. The report that the students prepared after participating in this event demonstrated that their understanding of the causes of violence was developed and that the need for community-wide mobilization and accountability became a clear theme in their discussions throughout the day (Deathe, 2001).

Program and Policy Development

The behavioral expectations and sanctions approach is a key component of any effort to reduce violence, and most schools now have a safe school document that outlines the pertinent policies and procedures. In Ontario, the Ministry of Education and Training provides guidelines and a template for these mandatory documents. These documents include principles of prevention and proactive strategies but focus mainly on acceptable codes of conduct, reporting procedures, and consequences of violent behavior. For schools with a more complex understanding of violence looking to balance the obedience approach with the skills development, the Program and Policy Development phase includes universal health promotion strategies. In the Thames Valley District School Board, an innovative health curriculum is currently being piloted in the grade 9 classes of three schools. This curriculum represents a marked departure from previous efforts in several ways. First, the effort is a collaborative one between researchers and the school board, and as such, teachers are involved with every step of development. A second innovative feature of this curriculum is that it approaches the prevention of violence and other high-risk behaviors by emphasizing the skills and awareness needed to make healthy relationship choices. Students engage in a discussion about their own boundaries and choices, are given the information needed to make good choices, and are then provided with many skill-building opportunities (such as role plays). In addition, there is discussion about how to intervene in situations of potential violence to overcome bystander apathy. This healthy relationship focus differs from other initiatives that emphasize naming violence and power and control issues above all other considerations. The current model is geared to engage adolescent boys (who tend to be alienated by the traditional power and control approach) and to focus on normative everyday violence so the issue is seen as relevant to all students. The third way that this curriculum differs from many other programs is in the universal implementation and curriculum format. The program was designed with close adherence to Ministry of Education standards and objectives so that it could replace the current health curriculum components of the mandatory grade 9 physical health education classes. There is the potential for the program to become an inherent part of every grade 9 program in the province, in contrast to being an "add on" program that depends on the enthusiasm and dedication of particular staff members. Although the pilot is still in the early stages, initial teacher and student responses have been very favorable.

Integration and Accountability

The integration part of the final stage refers to several types of integration. First, there needs to be collaboration among the different systems and stakeholders (e.g., parents, teachers, students, police, community agencies). Second, policies and programs need to be integrated with each other, and into the fabric of the school community. This type of integration means shifting away from addressing different types of issues as separate policies or one-day events (i.e., sexual harassment, bullying, racism, dating violence) and moving toward a comprehensive program to build a school climate of respect and positive relationships. One indication of the level of integration in the Thames Valley District School Board is the provision of a full-time violence prevention coordinator for the board, and a dedicated link on the school board website to update people about current violence prevention initiatives. These indications of an infrastructure to support violence prevention facilitate ongoing progress and convey a permanency and commitment to the violence prevention effort.

Integration also includes networking between schools and community agencies, and between schools that are at different points along the change continuum. The Forum Theatre program in the Thames Valley District School Board exemplifies the students' ability in a particular school to help raise awareness at other schools. This program consists of several troupes of talented student actors that travel to different schools and perform plays that have strong themes of violence and harassment. The plays were written as a collaborative effort between students and teachers, and are quite disturbing to watch. In the Forum Theatre approach, the play is performed start to finish once. Then, a teacher facilitator encourages people in the audience to put up their hand and yell "stop" when they see something they find unacceptable (e.g., an episode of bullying or harassment). When someone yells stop, the tableau freezes, and the person who stops the action replaces either the victim or the bystander (but not the perpetrator). The scene is then replayed with the person who intervened having the opportunity to effect a different outcome in the scene. The message arising from the Forum Theatre experience is a powerful one: everybody has the opportunity and the responsibility to stop violence, and without intervention, these scenes play out to disturbing conclusions. Discussion groups facilitated after the presentations find students disturbed by the scenes, but at the same time galvanized to take action to stop violence in their own schools.

The accountability facet of the final stage emphasizes that a commitment to violence prevention must be monitored. Clearly articulated spheres of responsibility throughout the whole system are necessary, and an annual report card outlining progress and remaining weaknesses should be implemented. For example, having violence prevention curricula that are credit courses is one way of attaching value to the endeavors of students. In keeping with the health promotion concept, schools that go beyond the bare minimum deserve extra recognition. In the Thames Valley District School Board, the violence prevention part of the website allows for this recognition to occur.

SUMMARY AND CONCLUSIONS

As the missing piece in our current educational approach, relationships, the "fourth R," are crucial both to understand violence and to counter violence in our schools. The Stage-Based School Change Model outlines a process through which schools can move toward a comprehensive approach. The paradigm's ability to match particular interventions to the needs of different stages along the change continuum underscores its usefulness.

The Stage-Based School Change Model approach to linking the needs of schools to specific types of intervention is merely the first step in customized intervention. The next step in this pursuit of flexible and responsive interventions will be the provision of a menu of options for different segments within a school body who may have unique requirements based on differences in culture, experience with violence, or gender. A careful needs assessment that identifies different groups within a school that may be at different stages along the readiness-to-act spectrum will lead to a multitiered approach that meets the prevention and intervention needs of each of these groups. Thus, a particular school might be ready for a universal promotion approach such as a curriculum but also have particular needs for interventions addressing students who have witnessed domestic violence, all offered in a way that is consistent with the cultural milieu of the school.

In closing, it is critical that we move beyond the obsession with identifying and punishing the "bad" youth in our schools to a comprehensive, well-integrated antiviolence approach. The youths who manifest extreme violence are those most vulnerable to the negative role models and attitudes that abound in our society, but they are by no means the only ones exposed to these detrimental messages. As noted by James Garbarino, the same risk factors that can reach a critical mass and result in young men's lethal violence are much more pervasive than would be inferred from the occurrence of tragedies like Columbine:

> The risk factors are there to be found in the more subtle forms of psychological maltreatment, in alienation from positive role models, in a spiritual emptiness that spawns despair, in adolescent melodrama, in humiliation and shame, in the video culture of violent fantasy that seduces many of the emotionally vulnerable, and in the gun culture that arms our society's troubled boys. (Garbarino, 1999)

It is clear that we have gone past the point of a "quick fix" for the problem of violence in schools. The struggle ahead requires sustained effort, thoughtful and proactive programming, and pervasive change in the climate and norms of our culture. Most of all, meaningful change requires adults to be challenged on their own behavior; each adult will have to choose to be part of the problem or part of the solution. There has been much discussion about schools becoming crucibles of violence and harassment; we must make a commitment to these same institutions becoming a crucible of change in promoting the critical importance of the neglected Fourth R, relationships.

REFERENCES

American Psychological Association. (1993). *Commission on violence and youth: Summary report.* Washington, DC: Author.

Burke, J. G., Carlson Gielen, A., McDonnell, K. A., O'Campo, P., & Maman, S. (2001). The process of ending abuse in intimate relationships: A qualitative exploration of the transtheoretical model. *Violence Against Women, 7,* 1144–1163.

Canadian Panel on Violence Against Women. (1993). *Changing the landscape: Ending violence—achieving equality.* Ottawa, Canada: Minister of Supply and Services Canada.

Day, D. M., Golench, C. A., MacDougall, J., & Beals-Gonzalez, C. A. (1995). *School-based violence prevention in Canada: Results of a national survey of policies and procedures.* Ottawa, Canada: Solicitor General Canada.

Deathe, A. (2001). *Report on violence prevention: Students' perspectives.* Report following the grade 11 initiative of the conference, Children Exposed to Domestic Violence: A Call to Action, London, Ontario.

Dwyer, K., Osher, D. & Warger, C. (1998). *Early warning, timely response: A guide to safe schools.* Washington, DC: U.S. Department of Education.

Elliott, D. S., Williams, K. R., & Hamburg, B. (1998). An integrated approach to violence prevention. In D. Elliott, B. Hamburg, & K. Williams (Eds.), *Violence in American schools.* Cambridge, UK: Cambridge University Press.

Erickson, W. H. (Chairman). (2001). *The Report of Governor Bill Owens' Columbine Review Commission.* Governor of Colorado.

Garbarino, J. (1999). *Lost boys: Why our sons turn violent and how we can save them.* New York, NY: The Free Press.

Levesque, D. A., Gelles, R. J., & Velicer, W. F. (2000). Development and validation of a stages of change measure for men in batterer treatment. *Cognitive Therapy and Research, 24,* 175–199.

National Film Board of Canada. (1999). *A love that kills.* Montreal, Quebec.

Pfeffer, J. (1993). Barriers to the advance of organizational science: Paradigm development as a dependent variable. *Academy of Management and Review, 18,* 599–620.

Porras, J. L., & Robertson, P. J. (1992). Organizational development: Theory, practice, and research. In M. D. Dunnette & L. M. Hough (Eds.), *Handbook of industrial and organizational psychology* (Vol. 3, pp. 719–740). Palo Alto, CA: Consulting Psychologists Press.

Prochaska, J. M., Prochaska, J. O., & Levesque, D. A. (2001). A transtheoretical approach to changing organizations. *Administration and Policy in Mental Health, 28,* 247–261.

Prochaska, J. O., & DiClemente, C. C. (1983). Stages and processes of self-change in smoking: Toward an integrative model of change. *Journal of Consulting and Clinical Psychology, 51,* 390–395.

Prochaska, J. O., & Velicer, W. F. (1997). The Transtheoretical Model of health behavior change. *American Journal of Health Promotion, 12,* 38–48.

Robins, S. L. (2000). *Protecting our students: A review to identify and prevent sexual misconduct in Ontario schools. Executive summary and recommendations.* Toronto, Ontario: Ontario Ministry of the Attorney General.

Stephens, R. D. (1998). Safe school planning. In D. Elliott, B. Hamburg, & K. Williams (Eds.), *Violence in American schools.* Cambridge, UK: Cambridge University Press.

Sudermann, M., & Jaffe, P. G. (1998). Preventing violence: School- and community-based strategies. In *Canada health action: Building on the legacy* (Vol. 3, *Settings and issues,* pp. 276–310). Sainte-Foy, Quebec: Editions MultiMondes.

Sudermann, M., Jaffe, P. G., & Schieck, E. (1996). *A.S.A.P.: A school-based anti-violence program—revised.* London, Ontario: London Family Court Clinic.

Van DeVen, A. H., & Poole, M. S. (1995). Explaining development and change in organizations. *Academy of Management Review, 20,* 510–540.

Wolfe, D. A., & Jaffe, P. G. (2001). Prevention of domestic violence: Emerging initiatives. In S. A. Graham-Berman & J. L. Edelson (Eds.), *Domestic violence in the lives of children: The future of research, intervention, and social policy.* Washington, DC: American Psychological Association.

Part IV

CONCLUSIONS

14

Future Directions in Ending Domestic Violence in the Lives of Children

Linda L. Baker, Alison J. Cunningham, and Peter G. Jaffe

This book has presented a series of chapters that share a central assumption. Children are best insulated from the effects of exposure to violence when their mothers can live safely and their fathers can function without violence. Our role in these efforts—abused women's advocacy and batterers' accountability and intervention—are most successful when part of an integrated, collaborative community response that includes emphasis on prevention, public education, and coordinated intervention.

At the Centre for Children and Families in the Justice System in London, Canada, we have struggled for almost 30 years with how most effectively to assist children and their parents when violence affects their homes. The children and adolescents often come through our doors disguised as young criminal offenders. More unmistakable, we see abused children reluctant to testify in court because of what the accused has done to them and often their mothers as well. We see children as pawns in custody battles when abusers' use ongoing power and control with ex-partners. We see adults who were traumatized as children, now seeking recognition and compensation through the civil courts. While we may do this work in southwestern Ontario, it is apparent from the geographic scope of the contributors to this volume that, no matter where the work is done, we all struggle with common issues.

It is helpful to remember that it was not so long ago that these assumptions were common:

- Children were not affected by the violence of their fathers unless they themselves were physically maltreated.
- Children who did not see acts of violence against their mothers were not exposed to and therefore were not affected by family violence.
- Men who abused, even killed, their wives were presumed to be good parents.

Consequences included these factors:

- One source of behavioral, social, and emotional problems was not recognized by therapists and others who intervened when child and adolescent problems came to light.
- The family courts were not sympathetic when women claimed their abusive ex-partners could pose a risk to the children, so the family courts could abet abusers' use of perpetual litigation as a form of ongoing abuse to undermine the nonabusive parent.
- Few if any violence-specific interventions were available for children.
- Researchers investigating the problems of children rarely if ever considered exposure to violence as a variable that might affect functioning.

When the consequences of exposure to violence go unappreciated and unstudied, the "system" may not effectively help mothers to minimize exposure to inappropriate role models and to seek safety and effective assistance for their children. This situation, in turn, places children at risk for physical maltreatment themselves.

We are currently undertaking a review of the literature on children exposed to violence, and in the course of this exercise we have uncovered well over 350 articles, reports, books, and chapters published since 1991.[1] Holden (1998) found only 56 empirical articles between 1975, when apparently the first two articles appeared, and 1995. So, there has been an explosion of interest in and attention to this issue over the past decade.

Today, several developments are apparent. While far from universal, they do indicate trends. For example:

- Across Canada, there are hundreds of group programs for children exposed to domestic violence.
- Children's mental health agencies routinely look for violence in the home as part of assessment and treatment planning.
- Family court judges are being educated about the dynamics of violence and the consequences for children.
- Child protection authorities in some jurisdictions regard family violence as a protection issue, and others see it as a risk factor.
- In some American states, exposing a child to violence is taken into account in the criminal sentencing process, sometimes as an aggravating factor in sentencing and sometimes as a separate offence.
- In Canada, evidence that an offender abused a spouse or child can be considered by the court as an aggravating factor in sentencing.
- Researchers commonly measure violence in the family in addition to other known correlates of poor outcomes in children.

The state of current knowledge was summarized in several chapters of this volume. Put briefly, research shows:

- Some children exposed to domestic violence may have an elevated likelihood of emotional, social, behavioral, and cognitive problems, compared with other children.
- Violence in the home is almost always associated with other risk factors, including child maltreatment.
- Some exposed children show no elevated rate of problems, or rates consistent with other risk factors in their lives (e.g., maltreatment, poverty, parental substance abuse).
- A number of factors may mediate, moderate, or interact with violence exposure to elevate the likelihood of problems or to create resiliency (e.g., age, sex, intelligence).
- The effects of violence exposure are expected to vary according to variables such as duration, severity, frequency, recency, and age of onset.
- Younger children are more likely to be exposed to violence, possibly an indication of the fact that rates of family violence are highest among young women and women with young children face the most challenges in leaving abusive marriages.

The sophistication of research has increased from small-scale studies of at-risk samples (e.g., children in shelters) to include prospective studies and general population surveys. Especially the large-scale epidemiological studies are yielding new light on the interplay of the many risk factors that characterize homes touched by violence.

INTERVENTIONS

Combining research-derived knowledge with that gained in the field informs interventions for children. Both specialized and general interventions have been modified as our understanding of violence exposure has expanded.

Child Protection Services

In many jurisdictions an ongoing and often heated debate is waged over the role of child protection services in violent families where the children are not themselves physically abused. Arguments by those who see violence exposure as a protection issue include:

- Exposure is a form of emotional abuse.
- These children are at elevated risk for maltreatment.
- The intervention could be helpful to the children.
- It is a powerful statement to the public and the abuser that domestic violence will not be tolerated.

The opposing viewpoint centers on a concern over penalizing the mother for "failure to protect" her children, thereby deflecting responsibility from the abuser himself. Clearly, a consensus on this issue will not be attainable in the near future.

Refocusing Existing Services

Mental health treatment for families has been modified over the years as service providers come to more fully appreciate how family violence can affect parenting and the emotional and behavioral functioning of children. This knowledge has informed both assessment and intervention.

Custody and Visitation Proceedings

Domestic violence is a relevant issue in custody and visitation disputes because:

- Abuse usually does not end with separation.
- There is a significant overlap between woman abuse and child abuse.
- Children with abusive fathers are exposed to inappropriate role models.
- An abusive ex-partner can undermine the nonabusive parent.
- Custody disputes can become perpetual litigation as a form of ongoing control.

In extreme cases, the children are at risk for abduction or even murder.

Specialized Services for Children

As we gain greater experience with interventions, it is often recognized that one size does not fit all. Increasingly, we are seeing gender-specific interventions for males and females, a tailoring of interventions to the developmental level of children and adolescents, and the modification of content and delivery style for the growing number of families who left their own countries for a new life in North America.

Coordination of Community Services and the Justice System

The tragically familiar conclusion of successive inquests and fatality reviews is that women and children are at risk for homicide when the criminal and family legal systems do not coordinate and share information or when the danger an abuser poses is not properly assessed. Many times, community agencies that provide services to women and children are in a better position to understand the risk. As these lessons are learned, communities are encouraging a more collaborative relationship among the many groups that have contact with abused women seeking safety. Safety planning is one of the most pervasive interventions provided to abused women, but this process does not always address the concerns a woman has about the safety of children on access visits. Collaborative training and program development can create a cross-pollination of skills to create a better service than any one professional group could provide in isolation.

Primary Prevention in Schools

Finally, one conclusion that is almost inevitably reached by most observers in this field is that family violence is a problem better prevented before it occurs than fixed after the damage is done. Educators across North America recognize their unique role as the setting through which all young minds will pass. Programs delivered in the schools—addressing bullying, harassment, family violence, and dating violence—can challenge pro-violence attitudes and help students develop healthy relationship skills. School-based efforts should not be limited to identifying and expelling the "bad kids."

WHAT LIES AHEAD

In the past 30 years, we have truly traveled many miles—but the journey continues. First, the above-listed advances are far from universal. Some communities have come farther down the road than others. We must ensure that all children and their parents benefit from what we have learned. Second, there are some new tasks upon which we must focus as we chart a course for the future.

Evaluate Groups for Children

The number of group programs for children exposed to violence has grown substantially in the past few years, including province-wide availability in British Columbia and Ontario, Canada. Such programs operate in a diverse array of settings that include child-protection agencies, women's shelters, and mental health agencies. To date, there have been few evaluations to document the overall effectiveness of these programs, let alone the relative effectiveness of different program models with different types of youth. This situation is easily traced to two factors: the infancy of the field relative to other more established interventions and the difficulty of attracting funding for rigorous evaluations. In consequence, the few published evaluations available are limited by problems such as methodologies that measure only pre- and post-changes in attitudes and knowledge acquisition, small samples, and lack of follow-up. Moreover, the best evaluations now available are efficacy studies conducted by the developers of the very programs they are evaluating, programs that are so resource rich that they are not readily transportable to field settings.

Many operational and evaluative questions remain unanswered:

- Are these programs effective in reducing symptoms associated with exposure?
- Are these programs effective in changing negative behaviors associated with exposure?
- Are violence-specific interventions more effective than general interventions?

- Are groups the most effective and efficient modality of intervention? For whom?
- Which type of child or adolescent benefits most? When?
- Which type of child or adolescent should not be placed in groups?
- Is effectiveness enhanced by concurrent mother groups?
- Is effectiveness enhanced by gender-specific or mixed-gender groups?
- Are there negative consequences of program participation? For whom?

The field is ready for an outcome evaluation that can answer these questions and is conducted by researchers other than the program's developers or deliverers. Indeed, expansion of programs should proceed cautiously until this step is taken.

Engage Men in Antiviolence Work

Men in general and fathers in particular have been marginalized from the antiviolence movement for a variety of good and bad reasons. Our collective efforts have focused primarily on women and children and assume that what is good for women is good for children. However, these facts remain true: (1) most violence is perpetrated by men, so they should help to fix the problem; (2) unless an abusive man is helped to change, he will probably start a new relationship and place other women and children at risk; and (3) some men can learn to be nonabusive.

While few men will leave batterers' treatment as feminists, the harm reduction concept applies if they have learned to be less toxic in their relationships. This work may require them to focus on their own childhoods.

We should think more about fathers and help them be involved as parents. The general public can be off put by the aggressive fathers' rights movement, men who are perceived as bitter misogynists. However, it is possible to reinforce the positive aspects of fatherhood, and there is a legitimate role for men as change agents. Additional research is also needed to make batterer typologies relevant for the field and to investigate which men have the most or least potential for change. The critical questions are: (1) What are the characteristics of men who are the least likely to change and who will continue to be a threat to women and children? and (2) Given this type of abuser, what is the most appropriate way to keep women and children safe through legal as well as community responses?

In addition, little is written about abusive men who do change. It is important to understand why and how this process occurs for them. Research could also be focused families where co-parenting relationships are sought by women despite histories of abuse.

Reach Out to Ethnocultural Groups

As our population becomes more culturally diverse, we must adapt both our methods of outreach and our intervention modalities to ensure that families new to the country do not face unreasonable barriers to human rights and services. These families can face considerable challenges in the months and years after arrival. Some have come from war-torn countries and suffer tremendous stress in the emigration process. Arriving in North America, they can face a bewildering array of challenges in acclimatizing to the culture and language.

Many abused women new to Canada and the United States are isolated in their homes, not just by the tactics of abusive men but by language, literacy, culture, the surveillance of in-laws and other extended family, and the absence of any means of learning about the services designed to help them. Our traditional models of intervention in woman abuse—shelters, criminal charges, empowerment advocacy, and divorce—may not be what these women want. Moreover, such interventions may elevate the risk to her and her children, even more than they do with Canadian and American women. Some women come from countries where honor killings are practiced with little if any sanction. Our model of woman abuse intervention, relying on women to self-identify and ask for help, may be culturally inappropriate in most cases. Moreover, assisting the few women who do come forward may be insufficient in the absence of interventions that address attitudes toward family violence in the larger family group and community.

Develop Research Instruments to Measure
Exposure/Experience of Violence

A significant impediment to conducting research on this topic is the lack of any valid and reliable measurement system for violence exposure. Requests for such a measure are one of the most frequent queries we receive at the Centre. Exposure varies in terms of variables such as age of onset, severity, duration, and frequency. Some children are themselves abused as well or witness the abuse of siblings. Some children are exposed to abuse by multiple father figures to whom they have varying degrees of attachment. An instrument that could capture all these dimensions, and weight them for importance, would help us move beyond the binary categorization of children as exposed or nonexposed. This, in turn, would assist greatly with research, including program evaluation.

Examine the Trajectory of Consequences in Prospective, Longitudinal Ways

With the results of several large-scale prospective studies of the general population now available, we are seeing how little we really know about any causal linkages between violence exposure and poor adjustment in children. This information, in turn, should be used to refine interventions. Many variables mediate, moderate, and interact with family violence to shape outcomes for children. It is especially important to learn more about resiliency and about youth with delayed onset of problems. Developmental sensitivity in our analysis is also important. In addition, we must consider how, or if, girls and boys are affected differently. There is also much that remains to be learned about the differential impact of violence exposure on different groups of youth, such as those in aboriginal families, ethnocultural minorities, new Canadians and Americans, and the disabled.

The perspectives of adult children who were exposed to violence against their mothers offer important insight into the effects of exposure to violence over time. These adults have had an opportunity to reflect on their experiences, as well as how the exposure to violence has influenced them, their relationships with parents, partners in their own marriage, and their children. Such insights may influence how we develop interventions.

Issues of Visitation

Visitation is an important issue in this discussion because routine interaction between fathers and children is necessary for meaningful involvement after separation. However, in families characterized by violence, this kind of interaction can be dangerous for women and children. More research is needed on the role of family courts and of visitation centers in attenuating or exacerbating the risk in these cases.

Document the Economic Costs of Violence Exposure

While there is insufficient information at present to calculate anything but a dramatic underestimate, placing a figure on the economic costs of family violence for children would encourage policymakers and legislators to recognize the fiscal burden of this largely hidden problem and the tangible benefits of effective prevention and intervention.

CONCLUSIONS

Over the past 30 years, we at the Centre for Children and Families in the Justice System have seen the devastating impact of domestic violence on families. Children and adolescents have come to our attention as young offenders, abuse victims, pawns in abusers' custody disputes, and court witnesses. Although the impact is unique for each child, the central themes are fear, anxiety, depression, anger, and withdrawal from school and community participation. Communities can no longer be passive bystanders to this harm. The contributors to this volume have voiced their own dreams on behalf of children growing up with domestic violence. These are dreams of a better understanding, more sensitive community responses, and genuine collaboration to end domestic violence. Our children deserve no less.

NOTES

1. A list of these references can be found at *www.lfcc.on.ca/CEFV_bib.html.*

Index